MW01407790

TO: Dear Mrs. Emily Panichi

Enjoy life!

Best wish

Quaqin Zh
趙
強
琴

1/27/2009

From Legend to Science

From Legend to Science

A History of Chinese Medicine

Ruan Jin Zhao, Ph.D.

VANTAGE PRESS
New York

The opinions and instructions expressed here in are solely those of the author. Each individual should seek the advice of his or her own physician before starting any new medical program.

Cover design by Polly McQuillen

FIRST EDITION

All rights reserved, including the right of
reproduction in whole or in part in any form.

Copyright © 2004 by Ruan Jin Zhao, Ph.D.

Published by Vantage Press, Inc.
516 West 34th Street, New York, New York 10001

Manufactured in the United States of America
ISBN: 0-533-14557-0

Library of Congress Catalog Card No.: 2003091305

0 9 8 7 6 5 4 3 2

To my family. They are my heart and soul.

Contents

Preface   ix

I—The Philosophical Basis of Chinese Medicine   1
    1. Early Theories on the Cause of the Disease   3
    2. Yin/Yang and the Five Elements   28
    3. Influences of the Three Great Philosophies   35

II—Diagnosis and Treatment   39
    4. Like Wood Floating on Water: Diagnosis Techniques in Chinese Medicine   41
    5. A Thousand Golden Formulas: The Development of Herbal Medicine   51
    6. Sea, River, Stream, Spring, Well: The History of Acupuncture and Moxibustion   75
    7. Preventative Medicine: The Cornerstone of Traditional Chinese Medicine   86

III—Clinical Medicine   91
    8. Internal Medicine   93
    9. Medicine for Women and Children   105
    10. Anatomy, Surgery, and Trauma   115

IV—Professional Standards   131
    11. A Note on Medical Ethics   133
    12. Medical Standards and the Education of Physicians   136

V—Traditional Chinese Medicine and Western Treatments 155
   13. HIV/AIDS 157
   14. Chronic Fatigue Syndrome 164
   15. Cancer 171
   16. Diabetes Mellitus 178
   17. Liver Diseases (Hepatitis B, Hepatitis C, Alcohol/Drug Induced Liver Damage and Liver Cirrhosis) 181
   18. Heart Disease 186
   19. Arthritis 189
   20. An Ideal Medical Model: Integrating Chinese Medical Philosophies & Ethics Into the Current Healthcare System 191

Appendix—A Chronology of Chinese Medicine 213
References 227

Preface

I began my study of Traditional Chinese Medicine at the age of fifteen. I did not originally want to be a doctor; I was fascinated by science and technology and had dreams of becoming a great engineer. But my parents decided that I should study medicine, so after high school (which in China is equivalent to American college), I began my studies in a school of Chinese Medicine. The first semester's courses on history and theory disappointed me, because they were more like literature or philosophy than science. One of my friends was enrolled in the college of pharmacology, and his courses sounded much more interesting: biophysics, analytical chemistry, advanced mathematics, and so on. I applied for a transfer and began trying to catch up on what I had missed during the first semester. By working very hard, I managed to pass the exams with fairly high scores and was formally admitted to the department of pharmacology the next semester. Two more semesters passed, and I was studying hard but still was not truly committed to becoming a doctor. How, I wondered, could these simple twigs and leaves cure disease? And how could this tiny acupuncture needle stop pain without any medication?

That summer I went back to my hometown for vacation to find my grandmother very ill. She was a beloved member of our family, and I was very close to her. She suffered from a high fever and could not eat or drink anything without vomiting. We took her to the nearest general hospital, but after ten days of treatment with both Western antibiotics and traditional herbal preparations, plus ice and alcohol washes to cool the fever, she did not improve. We were told that she was dying and that there was nothing else the hospital could do for her.

We brought grandmother home, and the whole family plunged into a deep sadness at the thought of losing her. Finally my mother said to me, "These barefoot doctors study for only a few months and then start treating people. You have studied medicine for two years now; you should do something to help your grandmother." I was started to hear this, because I had completely forgotten who I was in my grief at my dear grandmother's condition, and I never considered that I might be qualified to help her.

Quieting myself, I began to examine my grandmother. All her reflexes were normal. Her fever was still high (102–105F°), but she could recognize me. She still could not take anything by mouth—even water—without vomiting. I wondered how she would be able to take any herbal decoctions. I noticed that her tongue was very pale. Usually, with a high fever, we would expect to see a very red tongue. A pale color indicates something very specific: weak and deficient Qi (energy) of spleen and stomach. The treatment for this is to increase the spleen and stomach energy with warm medicine, rather than to clear heat, as had been tried at the hospital.

I remembered from my studies that there is a well-known formula for this condition. I looked it up in my textbook, took the prescription to the pharmacy, and mixed it up myself. I helped my grandmother sip it, spoonful by spoonful. We were surprised and pleased to see that she was able to take it without vomiting. She sipped it slowly until she had consumed about ten ounces. About thirty minutes later, her fever went down to 100°. An hour later, her temperature was normal, her mind was clear, and at the same time, many blisters appeared on her body, filled with a clear yellow fluid. I supposed that this was the toxin that had caused the fever. She fell into a deep sleep and woke four hours later complaining of hunger and pain on her skin. I directed my mother to prepare some well-cooked rice soup, which my grandmother was able to eat. A special herbal ointment was applied to her skin after the blisters had been drained. My grandmother quickly recovered, and is now eighty-five years old and quite healthy.

Her case astonished me, because neither I nor any of the doctors at the hospital expected her to recover. Because I had no experience at that time, I did not know what to expect from the treatment, but I realized then that this simple theory—Qi deficiency causes fever—came from real clinical practice and represented the essence of clinical experience gathered over thousands of years.

This experience with my grandmother changed my attitude completely. I realized how scientific Chinese medicine really is, and that the human body is much more sophisticated than any high-technology machine. I realized that there were many more mysteries to be explored. I went back to school the next semester with new enthusiasm and devoted myself wholeheartedly to the study of Traditional Chinese Medicine, eventually attaining a master's degree and a Ph.D. in Chinese medicine and cellular biology while participating in extensive clinical practice at Beijing University.

In 1993, I began practicing Chinese medicine in the United States. I was invited to lecture on the subject and noticed that many students were curious about the origins of Chinese medical techniques such as acupuncture and herbal pharmacology. I suggested a lecture series on the history of Chinese medicine to educate students on the historical basis of Chinese medicine and the extensive background of clinical experience from which the techniques are derived. Much of the material for this book is a result of those lectures.

My wife, Jing Lui, also graduated from Beijing University of Traditional Chinese Medicine. She studied Chinese Herbal

Pharmacology. We work together. Her dedication, work, and spirit helped me finish editing. Without her, there is no such book.

This book also could not have been written without the help and support of a fine person and a wonderful friend, Dr. Helga Wall-Apelt. Dr. Wall-Apelt practiced internal medicine for twenty-five years and then decided to explore new ways to help people. The techniques and theories of Traditional Chinese Medicine intrigued her, and she began studying with a view to future practice. Her dedicated spirit and optimistic attitude encouraged me to begin writing this book, and her collaboration on many aspects of the manuscript has been indispensable. I am grateful for her many contributions to this book as well as her enduring friendship.

Also, I am very grateful for my editor, Patricia Rockwood.

—Ruan Jin Zhao

I
The Philosophical Basis of Chinese Medicine

1
Early Theories on the Cause of Disease

Theories on the etiology of disease are as old as the observation of disease itself. Our information on the earliest Chinese theories comes mainly from four texts that were written sometime between 500 B.C. and 220 A.D. The most important of these is called *Huang Di Nei Jing* ("Internal Classic Cannon of the Yellow Emperor"). It was supposedly written by Huang Di, also known as the "Yellow Emperor," with the aid of the sage/physician Qi Bo, one of his ministers, and a group of other excellent physicians. The yellow emperor is one of the three "celestial emperors" who are credited with introducing the Chinese people to the essential sciences and other arts of civilization. Huang Di reigned 2698–2598 B.C. and is a brilliant character in Chinese medical history.

The *Nei Jing,* as it is commonly called, was most likely written not by the yellow emperor himself but by many authors over many years, who gradually compiled their observations and theories about disease and treatment. Indeed, the book itself refers to some twenty previous medical books (now lost). Later readers and practitioners of the art of medicine added to, edited, and revisited the work as they went along.

The text of *Huang Di Nei Jing* describes herbal medicine, acupuncture, moxibustion, and many other therapeutic modalities for the first time in Chinese literature. In the *Nei Jing* appear the first clear descriptions of the important theories of

Yin/Yang and the Five Elements that have shaped Chinese medical theory from the beginning (see chapter 2). The *Nei Jing* also covers theories concerning the viscera and bowels, channels and collaterals, pathology and the mechanisms of disease, diagnosis, differentiation of symptoms and signs, therapy, drugs and prescriptions, acupuncture and moxibustion, and the preservation of health. It thus codified the entire unique Chinese system of medical theory. This book is so thorough that it is still studied by students of Traditional Chinese Medicine.

The second important text in Chinese medical theory is called *Huang Di Ba Shi Yi Nan Jing* ("Yellow Emperor's Book of 81 Difficult Questions"). Written in a question-and-answer format, this important text is simple but precise; its title may have meant to convey the fact that medical theory is sophisticated and thus difficult to understand. Its author and publication date cannot be precisely fixed. One theory is that *Nan Jing* was written by Qi Yue Ren, a very famous clinician of his time who also was known as Bian Que (see p. 48). We do know that the work was completed some time before or during the Western Han Dynasty (206 B.C.–220 A.D.). In *Nan Jing*, eighty-one questions or topics are discussed, among them pulse diagnosis, the meridian/channel theory, viscera and bowel, disease pathology, acupoints, and acupuncture manipulation techniques.

Two other works from this period are *Zhou Li* and *Li Ji*, both of which offer some interesting theories concerning the relationship between weather and disease. These will be discussed in more detail later in this chapter.

The Idea of Balance

A theme that has pervaded Chinese medicine from the beginning has been the idea that physical and mental health depend on maintaining a balance between the person and the outside world and within the body itself. The Yin/Yang theory (described in more detail in chapter 2) is the foundation of this belief, but it is described with respect to the relationships between the various organs of the body in the *Nei Jing*.

According to the *Nei Jing*, the parts of the body are interrelated, and this relationship can be shown in physiology and in pathology. There is an exterior and interior relationship between the heart and small intestine, between the lung and large intestine, between the spleen and stomach, and between the liver and gall bladder. The heart governs the blood, blood circulation, and vessels and opens up to the tongue. The lung governs the skin and opens up to the nose. The spleen governs the musculature and the four extremities and opens up to the lips. The liver governs the tendons and opens up to the eyes. The kidney governs the bones and opens up to the ears. Every organ has its own responsibility, and all are required to cooperate with each other to maintain the physiological condition.

The balance among the organs is very important. One organ's problem can affect many other organs and tissues. Liver disease, for example, can affect the lungs, causing the patient to cough; a patient with a cough can thus be cured by regulating the function of the liver. It is also reasonable, under this theory, to treat a headache patient by not treating the head. Treating the human body as an organic, whole entity is a central concept in Chinese medicine that began with the *Nei Jing*.

The relationship between the body and the natural environment is another important fact of this idea of balance. It is emphasized repeatedly in the *Nei Jing* that the human body is an integral part of its surrounding natural environment. *Nei Jing* states that the human being lives "between heaven and earth," so the condition of his or her health will be affected by the climate, the changing of the seasons, and the geographical environment. It was believed very early on that the human body adapts to its natural environment. For example, the *Nei Jing* states: "Cold weather and less clothing make people produce more urine than perspiration; hot weather and thick clothing will produce more perspiration than urination." And again: "In the spring, head disease is common; chest and hypochondriac problems appear in the summer; diarrhea often occurs in long summer; malaria is common in autumn and arthritis and cold extremities are common and worse in winter." Other paragraphs describe how irregular weather can lead to attacks of epidemic plague.

The role of geographical conditions in human health is described in another part of *Nei Jing*: "On the east coast, there is a beach and sea, with fish and salt. People eat fish and other salty food. Fish makes heat accumulate inside the body and salt injures the blood and so the people are colored with black skin. They often suffer from carbuncles or abscesses. In the northern area, people live at a high elevation and fierce cold and ice. They stay outside and drink much milk, which makes the visceral bowels cold and distended." (This observation not only reflects the precise observation of an ancient doctor, but it also indicates that clinical practice was very common at that time.) In the *Nei Jing*, it was emphasized that for a doctor, knowledge of astronomy, geography, and natural science were as important as medical knowledge.

The Theory of Meridians

It was theorized in the *Nei Jing* that interactions among the various organs were made possible by linkage through a system of conduits rather like irrigation channels. Today these are known as meridians. These meridians connect all the organs into a unified system and provide them with nutrients (blood, energy, essence, and fluid). (The "essence" mentioned here is a very important substance for life. It may be comparable to what Western medicine calls hormones.) The theory of meridians is the basis of diagnosis, prognosis, and treatment.

Twelve regular (general) meridians/channels and eight extra channels were clearly documented in *Nei Jing*.[1] The twelve regular meridians, each connecting an extremity with internal organs, are: hand Tai Yin lung, hand Jue Y in pericardium, hand Shao Y in heart, hand Yang Ming large intestine, hand Shao Yao San Jiao (triple burner[2]), hand Tai Yang small intestine, foot Tai Yin spleen, foot Jui Yin in liver, foot Shao Y in kidney, foot Yang Ming stomach, foot Shao Yang gall bladder, and foot Tai Yang urine bladder. The eight channels are called Chong, Ren, Du, Dai, Yang Wei, Yin Wei, Yang Qiao, and Yin Qiao.[3] They were described in detail, and the precise route of each was clearly delineated with anatomical terminology.

Every channel is connected to its relative Zang (viscera) and extends to its Fu (bowels). In each channel, indications of disease are related to its organ and its route. For example, the Hand Shao Yin Heart meridian begins in the heart and extends in one direction to include the esophagus and eye, and in the other direction to include the lung, small intestine, arm and hand. Points on this meridian are indicated mainly in diseases of the cardiovascular system (such as angina, irregular heartbeat, etc.) and other disorders such as epilepsy, insomnia, and certain mental disorders such as psychoses and neuroses.

The Influence of Weather on Disease

During the Zhou Dynasty (1122–249 B.C.), great strides in agriculture, astronomy and the calendar arts, religion, science, and culture greatly facilitated the development of the medical arts as practitioners began to think more abstractly, and experimental science gradually grew out of practical technique. As more was learned about the effects of weather on crops, for example, it was recognized that the natural environment could also have an effect on the human body.

Several early texts discussed this theory. The book *Zhou Li* ("Rituals of Zhou Dynasty") observed that particular weather conditions can cause particular diseases. In the springtime, states the author, headaches are common; in summer, itching; in autumn, malaria may be widespread. Coughs and asthma appear during winter. In addition, unseasonable weather was deemed responsible for illness. The book *Li Ji* ("Record of Rites") suggests that if there is an autumnlike wind during the early spring, there will be outbreaks of severe epidemic disease; if the weather conditions are hot and summerlike in late spring, there will be more sickness.

During this period, many diseases were recognized by observation and experience. Terms such as fever, coma, edema, normal childbirth, and infertility appear for the first time in history. Actual disease names such as hemorrhoid, carbuncle, cellulitis, paralysis, malaria, mania, epidemic disease are found, as well as diseases recorded by symptom, such as swelling, drum distention, sore throat, vomiting, and deafness.

The Six Evil Qi

In 541 B.C., Yi He, a famous doctor of the province of Qin, developed a theory of pathology to explain how "Six Evil Qi" had caused a disease suffered by the king of Jin state, as well as many other diseases. "There are six Qi[4], he wrote, "which produce five odors and express themselves in five colors, and sound five tones, under hyperactive conditions to cause disease. The six are Yin, Yang, Feng (Wind), Yu (Rain), Hui (gloom), and Ming (brightness).... There are four seasons, and five stages to the sequence (spring, summer, long-summer, autumn, and winter). Cold disease," he continued, "occurs with over Yin, heat disease with over Yang, sickness in the extremities with over Wind, stomach problems with too much Rain, confusion of the mind with excessive Gloom and humidity, and heart disease with the strong radiation (brightness)."

Yi He's conclusions about heat, cold, over Yin, and over Yang were the primary basis for the later theory of six exogenous pathogenic factors that lead to the imbalance of Yin and Yang (see p. 30). His observations on other relationships—such as diseases of the extremities and wind, gastroenteritis and excess humidity, or rain—also are ingenious.

Etiology and Symptom Description

By the time of the Sui Dynasty (590–618 A.D.), tremendous progress had been made in the exploration of the sources and symptoms of disease. About 600 A.D., the definitive treatise in this field was written by Cao Yuan Fang and others: *Zhu Bing Yuan Hao Lun* ("Etiology and Manifestation of Many diseases"). *Zhu Bing Yuan Hao Lun* summarizes clinical experiences up to the time of the Jin Dynasty and discusses 1,039 symptoms and syndromes. Etiology, clinical manifestations, diagnosis, and prognosis were described in detail. Great emphasis was placed upon recommending dietary and other lifestyle requirements for the patient to adopt after the disease had been cured.

The principal contribution of this book was its wide-ranging and detailed description of each disease. The primary syndromes were listed for conditions such as stroke, arthritis, Xu Lao (fatigue syndrome), common cold/flu, chicken pox, cholera, malaria, dysentery, edema, jaundice, diabetes, athlete's foot, gastritis, hemorrhoids, and carbuncles. Gynecological and obstetrical problems were included, such as diseases during pregnancy and the postnatal period (five categories in the latter alone), complications during delivery, irregular menstruation, profuse vaginal discharge, breast abscess, and morning sickness.

Cao Yuan Fang also included the etiology of each disease based upon his own clinical research. He theorized that some infectious diseases are caused by exogenous evil substances, that they have contagious properties, and that they can be prevented by the administration of appropriate medicine. His observational skill was helpful in connection with parasitic diseases. For instance, he pointed out that there are worms in scabies, and that they could be picked out with a needle. The thread worm infection, he said, was related to eating raw beef.

In the area of allergic disease, he discovered that a reaction to lacquer, for example, was constitutional. *Zhu Bing Yuan Hao Lun* also precisely recorded some endocrine and nutritive diseases. It described, for example, the diabetic's symptoms of thirst and profuse urination, even mentioning complications such as neuropathy and carbuncles. All of these observations were based on abundant clinical observation.

Theories About the Flow of Energy

Two new philosophical schools appeared during the Song Dynasty (960–1279). One was named Li Xue ("Theoretical Principle"), and the other Xin Xue ("New Theory"). Both of these affected medical theory. Li Xue claimed that there is a principle, which, on its own, will generate Qi (vital energy as expressed in two forms—Yin and Yang). According to this theory, the five elements and this energy (Qi) are found in all things on earth, and the human body is a combination of this principle and Qi. The Li school's teachings concerning the flow of energy affected medical theory by directing it away from superstition toward exploration of the natural rules of the human body. Due to the influence of this theory, the Song government went so far as to issue a "calendar of Yun," which informed the populace of the possibilities of epidemics and appropriate preventative and therapeutic measures. Li Xue has engendered much debate in the medical field ever since; part of it makes sense, in that applying it can often predict what will happen with a person's health, and part of it can clearly be seen to be nonsense because it cannot possibly be comprehensive.

The Xin Xue theory claimed that everything in the world consists of, and is derived from, the five elements. It claimed also that a dichotomy is inherent in life forms (opposing magnetic poles), and that, though these are opposites, they are dependent upon each other—somewhat like the relationship between Yin and Yang. Further, it advised that change is brought about through certain intrinsic factors and will. Although this theory is not in practice today, it served an important purpose in stimulating later academic thought in the field of pathology.

The Theory of Three Factors Causing Disease

Theories about the etiology of disease had been evolving since the *Nei Jing*. After the Tang Dynasty (618–906 A.D.), Wang Bing added nineteen principles of pathology to those existing in the *Nei Jing*. Song and Yuan Dynasty doctors also made strides in this area. In 1171 A.D., Chen Yan (Wu Ze) wrote a book in which he outlined the theory of three factors causing disease. These three factors were: (1) internal factors, such as emotional disturbances from too much joy, anger, anxiety, "thinking too much," grief, or fright. This factor comes from the internal organs and appears on the extremities (outside); (2) exogenous factors, including climatic conditions, such as wind, cold, summer heat, damp, dryness, and fire. Such a factor starts from the outside and affects the channel and collateral (very small channel), then goes into the internal organs; (3) miscellaneous factors, including improper diet, animal attacks, poisonous insects, drowning, and trauma/accident. This classification was based on Zhang Zhong Jing's etiologic theory (see below). The related syndrome, clinical manifestations, and any special comments were given for each category.

Zhang Zhong Jing—a Pioneer in the Study of Febrile Disease (includes illustration of Zhang)

Shang Han Za Bing Lun ("Treatise on Febrile Disease caused by Cold and the Miscellaneous Diseases") has been called the first book on internal medicine. Its author was Zhang Zhong Jing, respectfully known as "the sage of medicine." Zhang was born in Henan Province. It is not known precisely when he lived, but it was approximately from 150 to 219 A.D., at the end of the East Han Dynasty.

Civil war and epidemic plagues were rampant during that time, attested to by the original preface to the *Treatise on Febrile Disease,* in which Zhang states that two-thirds of the two hundred original members of his family had died within the previous ten years of a severe infection. This personal tragedy gave Zhang Zhong Jing the impetus to research and explore the dreaded disease, and to write this great clinical medical book.

For a short time after its publication, *Shang Han Za Bing Lun* was lost due to war. What we have now was reedited during the Western Jin (265–316 A.D.) and Southern Song (1127–1279) Dynasties as two books known as *Shang Han Lun* ("Treatise on Febrile Diseases Caused by Cold") and *Jin Gui Yao Lue Fang Lun* ("Synopsis of Prescriptions of the Golden Chamber"). Both books are regarded as important classics of Traditional Chinese Medicine. In his writing, Zhang Zhong Jing summed up his own clinical experience and established a system of diagnosis and treatment based on an overall analysis of symptoms and signs. Because of this bridge between fundamental theory and clinical practice, his book has remained a vital text in Traditional Chinese Medicine.

The Contributions of *Shang Han Za Bing Lun*

After thorough study of the theories of febrile diseases espoused in the "Canon of Medicine" (*Nei Jing*), Zhang Zhong Jing scrutinized the whole progressive procedure of exogenous (caused by external organisms) disease. Assessing the invaded (affected) channel and its collateral, the functional condition of internal organs, the patient's resistance energy, and preexisting health problems (if any), he was able to ascertain the general characteristics of the disease. He used the differentiation syndrome according to Six Channels (see below) as his principle to distinguish the febrile disease caused by cold, relying upon the relationship between the collaterals and internal organs.

Zhang's book discusses miscellaneous internal diseases, such as malaria, stroke, lung disease, heart disease (congestive heart failure, angina), diabetes, jaundice, vomiting blood, diarrhea, and so on. It also examines many gynecological problems, such as premenstrual syndrome, morning sickness of pregnancy, and postpartum disease. Some surgical diseases also were mentioned, such as appendicitis and cellulitis. Also included were several resuscitative techniques, such as manual respiration in cases of strangulation.

The principle of differentiation of the syndrome according to Zang Fu (internal organs) was established by Zhang, and it has proved to be precise in syndrome classification, differentiation, diagnosis, and treatment. Differentiation principles established by Zhang are still used in clinical practice. "Differentiation of syndrome" refers to the approach used by doctors to analyze the patient's symptoms in order to make a correct diagnosis and prescribe suitable treatment. The method used most often in current clinical practice is the "Eight Principles," which are Yin-Yang, exterior-interior, excess-deficiency, and cold-heat. Zhang emphasized both principle and flexibility in differentiation and treatment, creating the maxim, "Observe the pulse and syndrome, determine which channel and organ was affected, and then follow the syndrome to establish your therapeutic principle."

Zhang Zhong Jing was the first doctor to describe the pathogenesis theory of three factors: internal, exogenous, and traumatic injury. He also described the eight therapeutic principles: diaphoresis (sweating), used to expel external pathogens; purgation (bowel movement), used if the pathogen is internal; enphoresis (vomiting), if the pathogen is in the upper body; harmonization (balance); clearing (reducing the heat of the body); tonifying (used if patient is very weak and energy-deficient); and transforming (digestion).

In his text, Zhang also discussed the principles of pharmacology, recording 262 formulas and expanding methods of administration to include evaporation, ear drops, nasal drops, ointment, and rectal and vaginal suppositories. Most of the formulas he listed are still considered efficacious, such as Bai Hu Tang (white tiger decoction) for meningitis, Bai Tou Ong Tang (pulsatilla decoction) for dysentery, Yin Chen Hao Tang (evergreen artemisia decoction) for jaundice, Shen Qi Wan (kidney energy pill) for diabetes, and Gua Luo Xie Bai Tang (trichosanthes fruit and macrostem onion decoction) for congested heart/heart attack.

Shang Han Za Bing Lun marked a drastic advance in Chinese medicine by integrating medical theory with clinical practice, laying a solid foundation of treatment and diagnosis based on overall analysis of symptoms and signs.

Many medical theories and therapies were born during the Song and Yuan Dynasties (960–1368 A.D.) for several reasons: changing ideology, which affected medical thinking, and the recognition of new diseases. Credit for most of the innovations during this period must be given to two twelfth-century schools of medical theory—He Jian and Yi Shui—and, in the fourteenth century, the Jin Yuan Famous Four Doctors (Liu Wan Su, Zhang Cong Zheng, Li Gao and Zhu Zhen Heng).

Fire and Heat Theory

Liu Wan Su (1120–1200) gave himself the title Tong Xuan Chun Shi. ("One Who Knows the Mystery of This World"). Born in He Jian, Hebei Province, he was thrice offered official positions by the emperor of the Jin Dynasty. He refused, however, preferring to practice medicine. He was best known for challenging old theories and replacing them with new ones if they did not hold up under scrutiny. His research and subsequent contribution to medical science were legendary, as attested to by the many memorials in his honor.

Doctor Liu Wan Su did not agree entirely with the fashionable theory of the day, that all disease was a product of the weather and environmental conditions. While not disagreeing that weather and such were causes of many diseases, he suggested that in addition to this, disease occurred due to lack of care. His principal theory was called Fire and Heat, and was based on his assumptions that febrile disease caused by cold has a close relationship with the pathogens in fire and heat.

Traditionally, as recorded in *Nei Jing*, Chinese doctors had held that fire and heat were in second place on the list of the six exogenous pathogens (see p. 8). However, Dr. Liu reasoned, the other pathogens—wind, damp, dryness, and so on—could be transformed into fire and heat during the course of the disease, as well as cause interior wind and dryness. Therefore, he concluded, all six were based upon fire and heat.

Relying on his theory, Liu Wan Su preferred the heat-clearing therapeutic principle, using cold-property herbs when treating febrile diseases. This theoretical practice he later named the Cold and Cool School. When prescribing hot-property herbs, depending on the differentiation of syndrome, he utilized aconite, dry ginger root, cinnamon bark, and nutmeg.

Zang Fu Theory

Zhang Yuan Su (1151–1234), also known as Jie Gu, was born in Hebei Province. His doctrine was named the Yi Shui School, after the county in which he was born. A precocious child, he passed the national examination for government service when he was only eight years old. At the age of twenty-seven, while sitting for further examination, he used a prohibited word (perhaps the emperor's name); as a result, he was dismissed from government service. After much study, he entered the medical field and created for himself a highly regarded position. A neighbor and friend of Liu Wan Su, he once treated and cured his colleague's febrile disease.

Unfortunately, among his many medical writings, only three have come down to us. He superseded the medical theories of Zhang Zhong Jing and developed his own pattern for the use of herbal medicine, basing it on differentiation between the excess, deficiency, cold, and heat of the "Zang Fu" (internal organs) to make an accurate prognosis of disease. He also classified herbs into four categories: warm, cool, tonifying, and reducing. For example, he explained the lung's pattern in this way:

Lung

Excess Syndrome

>
> To reduce the sun (kidney)—Alisma tuber, Epidium seed
> To drain the damp—Pinella tube, Tangerine peel
> To clear the fire—Gypsum, Anemarrhena rhizoma
> To open the blockage—Bitter orange peel, Apricot seed

Deficiency Syndrome

> To tone the mother (spleen)—Ginshen root, Cimicifuga rhizoma
> To moisturize the dryness—Ophiopogon root, fritillary bulb
> To construct the lung—Black plum, Schisandra fruit

Heat Syndrome

> To clear the lung's heat—Scutellaria root, Anemarrhena rhizoma

Cold Syndrome

> To warm the lung's cold—Cloves, Coltsfoot flower
> To disperse the superficial cold—Ephedra, Perilla leaf

This general pattern was a great aid in exercising the differentiation of syndromes in clinical practice.

Another outstanding achievement of Zhang Yuan Su was in pharmacology. He developed the channel-entered theory and messenger medicine formula. "Channel-entered" means that each medicine has its own preferred organ or channel. A "messenger medicine" refers to one component in a formula that targets the specific channel needing treatment and leads the other herbal properties to that area. These principles, along with his discovery that a single herbal medicine can have differing effects on various parts of the body, led to the establishment of many effective formulas and helped consolidate some of the prevailing theories of the time.

The Purgative School

Zhang Cong Zheng (1156–1228) was born in Lan Kao, Henan Province. He was close friends with two other well-known doctors, Ma Zhi Ji and Chang Zhong Ming. Together they wrote the book *Ru Men Shi Qin* ("Parental Care According to the Way of Confucius"). Because his emphasis was on expelling pathogens (thereby restoring body balance and permitting the patient's natural resistance to bring about recovery), his was known as the Purgative School. Extending Liu Wan Su's theory about exogenous pathogens, such as wind, cold, heat, damp, dryness, and fire, he included pathogens from improper food. His conclusion was that all of these factors were foreign to the body and should be expelled. His method was based on diaphoresis (sweating), vomiting, and purgation (bowel movement).

The principles were outlined thus: If the pathogen is located cutaneously (on the surface of the skin), a diaphoretic should be used. If the cause is wind, and phlegm and undigested food are accumulating in the upper body (Shang Jiao), inducing vomiting is the correct method. If the pathogen is of cold, damp, or heat in origin and affecting the lower part of the body (Xia Jiao), purgation would be the appropriate method.

Zhang Cong Zheng outlined specific treatments for his procedures. For diaphoretics, he recommended moxibustion, evaporation, bathing, acupuncture, and massage. Into the vomiting category, he also included draining the saliva, expectorants, and inducing tears and sneezing. Also he delineated the uses of purgation as inducing menstruation, birth, and mother's milk, breaking up masses, diuretics, and expulsion of gas.

Expanding upon the application of tonification in clinical practice, he added other medicines to the commonly used ginseng and astragalus root (still used in clinical practice today for this purpose). Previously, tonification meant only rebuilding the body's energy. Zhang expanded the term to include expelling pathogens in this indirect manner.

Recognizing the detrimental effects of an unstable social environment and its disturbance upon physical and emotional health, Zhang developed an early type of psychiatric therapy. As part of the treatment, he urged consideration of individual physical constitution and geographic region.

Spleen and Stomach Theory

Li Gao (1180–1251) was born into a large affluent family in Zhen Ding, Hebei Province. Shaken by his mother's death as a result of treatment by an unqualified doctor, he was moved to study medicine himself and eventually became a great doctor. Among his contributions to medicine was his development of the Yi Shui school of thought.

Simply said, Li Gao enhanced the differentiation theory according to the Zang Fu (see p. 16). He clearly distinguished external from the internal diseases and established his unique and practical spleen and stomach theory, which laid the responsibility for many diseases on disorders of the spleen and stomach. Because he was an expert in the technique of warming and toning the spleen and stomach, his was named the "Tonify Earth School."

Since the *Nei Jing*, stomach Qi (energy) had been thought of as the vital life source and original energy of the human body. "Life means the existence of stomach Qi, death means there is no stomach Qi," said the *Nei Jing*. Li Gao enlarged upon this definition, pointing out that the spleen and stomach are the source of Yuan Qi (original vital energy). He postulated that when Yuan Qi is decreased and there is deficiency due to injury of the spleen and stomach, disease will result.

Li Gao concluded that there were three causes of spleen and stomach disorders: (1) improper diet, including cold and bad food, becoming overly hungry, and overindulgence; (2) fatigue/overwork; and (3) emotional extremes. For example, emotional disturbances, such as too much joy, anger, grief, anxiety, and fear, can increase the heart fire, which will exhaust and burn out Yuan Qi, resulting in the disorder of the spleen and stomach. This pathological theory led Li Gao to choose the tonification of spleen and stomach energies as the focus of his treatments. He added some flexible therapies to increase relatively the Shang (Upper), Zhong (Middle), and Xia (Lower) Jiao in clinical practices. The series of three therapeutic principles was based on Li Gao's constant theme of regulating the spleen and stomach and elevating the clear Yang. He created many effective medicinal formulas according to this basic principle.

Work on spleen and stomach dysfunction led to further discoveries, such as the efficacy of warm herbal medicine in the treatment of high fever. A significant limitation of Li's theory is that he emphasized the importance of stomach Yang and neglected stomach Yin. Several hundred years later, during the Qing Dynasty, this shortcoming was corrected by a doctor named Ye Tian Shi (see p. 24).

Yin Syndrome

Wang Hao Gu (1200–1300) was born in Zhao County, Hebei Province, and became a professor of history and Chinese literature before deciding to take up medical practice. It is unclear whether he was a classmate or a student of Li Gao, but it is certain that he learned from the clinical experience of Li, became a great doctor in the Yi Shui School, and authored many books, all of which are treasured documents in Traditional Chinese Medicine.

Wang is best known for his work on the Yin Syndrome, which is difficult to diagnose, because, as a deficiency syndrome, it can easily be confused with heat and fire syndrome. He listed its symptoms: thirst, cough, fever, constipation, dysuria, deep and thin pulse, or floating and wiry pulse, and no energy. Due to the weakness of the spleen and kidney, pathogens can easily invade the body. In treatment, Wang emphasized the tonification of the kidney. He wrote: "As soon as the kidney Qi is strong, the skin and muscles will be strong enough to resist the devil pathogen."

In clinical practice, Wang Hao Gu matched febrile diseases caused by cold with miscellaneous diseases and, using the six-channel differentiation principle for internal disease (see p. 13), came up with a cure. The long-term advantages of his success was that it introduced flexibility in dealing with complex diseases in clinical practice, which, in turn, augmented treatment formulas. Because he considered the cold and heat in the San Jiao (triple burner) and in blood when differentiating the location of disease, and used this to select the medical formula, he enlarged the scope of the differentiation by syndrome to include the San Jiao and Wei Qi Ying Xue (four stages; see p. 24).

Wang Hao Gu's work had some shortcomings. While he emphasized observation and pulse taking in clinical diagnosis, he neglected the inquiry and olfactory techniques. In treatment, he paid much attention to the Kidney Yang but neglected the kidney itself.

Theory of Primary Fire

Zhu Zhen Heng (1281–1358) was born in Yi Wu County, Zhejiang Province, during the Yuan Dynasty. Because his family had lived near Dan Xi for generations, he took the title of Dan Xin. In his thirties, spurred on by the death of a relative who had been maltreated by a physician, Zhu began to study medicine. As his reputation grew, the famed doctor Luo Zhi Di took him under his wing and imparted to him all of his knowledge.

At age thirty-six, Zhu took his first step on what was to become a major pathway in his life. He became a disciple of the Li Xue school of philosophy, founded by Zhu Xi. The tutelage of the school's great thinkers and scholars was to have far-reaching effects on his work, influencing even his medical research. His ethics and professional technique were most appreciated by his local patients as well as those he treated during his travels to southern cities.

The theory of Xiang Huo (Primary Fire) assigns Xiang Huo the role of original life force, which maintains the human being's physiological condition. This would mean that all the organs function because of Xiang Huo. However, Zhu theorized, hyperactivity of the Xiang Huo can cause pathological damage by burning out the original Yin (essential substance). Manifestations of this would be dizziness, fever, lumbar-region soreness, confusion, difficulty in concentration, irritability, and pain. His treatment, then, was to tonify Yin with a nourishing Yin and decrease the fire medicine. Thus he arrived at his doctrine named "Yang Yin Pai," meaning "Nourishing Yin School." Other treatments he developed were aimed at preventing Xiang Huo hyperactivity, protecting the Original Yin, and controlling sexual desire (because it was believed to exhaust original energy).

In clinical practice, he was against what he considered overuse of the pungent and dryness medicine advocated by Ju Fang without differentiation. His dictum was: "The Yang always will be overactive; the Yin will always be deficient."

Theory of Li Qi ("Epidemic Pathological Evil")

Wu You Xing, also called You Ke, lived sometime during the seventeenth century. He was born in Wu County, Jiangsu

Province, and lived through a time of plague. Saddened by the suffering around him, he started his research, basing much of it on observation made during clinical practice. In writing *Wen Yi Lun* ("Treatise on Epidemic Diseases"), which was published in 1642, he established his Li Qi theory. In essence, it presaged the discovery of bacteria some two hundred years later.

The main points are:

1. Yi Bing (epidemic disease) is caused by Li Qi, which is something other than the usual pathogens of wind cold, summer heat and damp.
2. Li Qi is a substance. It can be controlled by medicine.
3. Li Qi invades the body from the mouth and nose. Whether it will cause disease depends upon its toxicity and the body's resistance.
4. Li Qi has many variations, each of which can affect different organs.
5. Li Qi that causes disease in animals cannot affect human beings, and vice versa.
6. Measles, chicken pox, small pox and some abscesses (infections), also are caused by Li Qi.

The Theory of Wen Bing

Febrile disease caused by heat (Wen Bing) evidences general symptoms comparable to all febrile diseases, including both the infectious and noncontagious ones. Wen Bing was first mentioned in the *Nei Jing*. Its etiology was nebulous; Wen Bing was listed under the category of Shang Han (febrile disease caused by cold), which category also included "damp and heat syndrome" and "heat syndrome."

During the Han Dynasty, Zhang Zhong Jing described the initial symptoms of Wen Bing (see p. 24). He established a basis for further exploration by creating the "clearing heat" formula.

During the Jin Dynasty, Wang Shu classified varieties of Wen Bing according to their descriptions in the *Nei Jing*—such as Wen Nue (malaria), Feng Wen (wind heat syndrome), Wen Du (heat toxicity syndrome), Wen Yi (heat infectious syndrome), and Shu Bing (summer heat syndrome). The Sui Dynasty's Cao Yuan Fang described the thirty-four syndromes of Wen Bing and especially pointed out its contagious characteristics. In the Tang Dynasty, many formulas for clearing heat were reworked.

During the Song and Yuan Dynasties, Wen Bing was separated from the Shang Han category. Liu Wan Su clearly pointed out that pungent and warm medicines are contraindicated during the initial stage of Wen Bing. He invented a pungent and cool method both to release the exterior and clear the interior, while tonifying the Yin and clearing heat. His formula was called Shuang Jie San. In the early days of the Ming Dynasty, Wang Li concurred that Wen Bing is much different from Shang Han. Wen Bing was caused by interior heat, he said, and the clearing heat principle should be used.

Follow-up work was done by other doctors in later centuries. One of the most influential was Ye Gui. Ye Gui (1667–1746), also called Tian Shi, learned medicine from his father and grandfather, both of whom were doctors. He specialized in infectious diseases, and his work was collected and edited for publication by his student, Gu Jing Wen, as Ye Gui devoted his time to the practice of medicine and had no time to write. The book was entitled *Wen Re Lun* and included the following main points about Wen Bing:

1. The general principle of transmission and progression of Wen Bing: when the pathogen invades the body, it goes first to the lung then reverses back to the pericardium.

2. The four stages in the progression of Wen Bing by which it can be treated effectively: Wei (defensive level), Qi (energy level), Ying (nutrient level), and Xue (blood level).

When the pathogen is in the Wei stage, diaphoresis is the therapeutic principle. When in the Qi stage, clearing heat (Qi) is indicated. If the pathogen goes into the Ying stage, it is still sometimes possible to return to the Qi stage by clearing Ying's heat. But when the pathogen goes into the Xue stage, the blood must be quickly cooled.

3. The development of a framework for the differentiation of Wen Bing: several diagnostic techniques were described, such as observing the tongue, testing the teeth, and differentiating the rash.

Xue Xue (1681–1770), who lived in Wu County, Jiangsu Province, became proficient in treating Shi Re (Damp Heat) disease and wrote a book about it, discussing its pathogenesis, clinical manifestations, progression, prognosis and recommended therapy.

Wu Tang (1758–1736) lived in Hui Ying, Jiangsu Province. His book, titled *Wen Bing Tiao Bian* ("Differentiation of Causes in Febrile Disease Caused by Heat"), was published in 1798. It was based on the experiences of Ye Tian Shi and used Wu Tang's own differentiation system of San Jiao (Triple Burners). He theorized that after the Wen Bing enters through the mouth, it spread to the stomach, and when entering through the nose, it spreads to the lung. If Wen Bing is not treated properly, it can invade more deeply in several ways: affectation of the lung can transfer to the pericardium, or the Shang (upper) Jiao syndrome can transfer to the middle Jiao, then to the lower Jiao.

Wen Bing was classified into nine syndromes: Fang Wen (wind-heat), Wen Re (warm-heat), Wen Yi (warm epidemics), Wen Du (heat toxicity), Shu Wen (summer-heat), Shi Wen (damp-heat), Qiu Zao (autumn dryness), Dong Wen (winter-heat), and Wen Nue (heat malaria). He further categorized the therapeutic principle for Wen Bing into Qing Luo (clear the collateral), Qing Ying (clear nutrimental) and Yu Yin (culture the Yin). According to these principles, he created many effective medicinal formulas. He also augmented the applications for several patent medicines.

Wang Shi Xiong (1808–1866), also known as Meng Ying, was born in Qian Tang, Zhejiang Province and moved to Shanghai when he was forty-two. He wrote many books, one of which focused on the etiology and clinical manifestations of cholera. He discovered that dirty drinking water was the medium through which the disease was spread. He collected ancient descriptions of Wen Bing from the *Nei Jing* and *Shang Han Lun*, information from the contemporary works on Wen Bing, and his own opinions and theory in this book, making it one of the most complete works on the subject. Of special note was the new classification of Wen Bing into two types. The first is Fu Qi (hidden pathological factor), in which there are no clinical symptoms at the time the pathogens invade the body (an example would be the dormant stage of HIV infection when no symptoms show). The second is Xin Fa (with symptoms appearing immediately upon infection).

As is apparent from the above discussion, most of the doctors active in research on Wen Bing were from the Jiangsu and Zhejiang regions. At that time the area was well developed culturally and economically. Travel was easy there, with river transportation accommodating a large travel population, which helped to spread the disease. These factors prompted doctors to study Wen Bing, including its theory as an independent subject in Chinese medicine. It complemented the Shang Han Theory, allowing a clearer understanding of and more effective treatment options for infectious diseases.

Notes

1. In 1970, some early medical books were discovered in a Han Dynasty (206 B.C.–220 A.D.) tomb in Changsha, Huan Province, in which eleven channels are described. One of the contributors of *Nei Jing* thus must have added the twelfth channel.

2. Especially outstanding in the book *Nan Jing* is the description of the triple burner (San Jiao) and Ming Men (spirit, gate, or life gate). "Triple burner" was the name originally given to the three parts of the human torso cavities. In this text it was given a more exact meaning; it was thought to be a separate organ with its own function, that of serving as a passageway for water and "original energy" (Yuan Qi). Original energy is the life source that we get from our parents and which is stored in the Ming Men (spirit gate or life gate). The place for storing the life source was thought to be located just above the right kidney—the exact location of what we now know to be the adrenal gland, a very important source indeed for the vitality of life.

3. The eight extra meridians have no specific pathways in the body, but they have these three important functions: to govern the functions of the twelve regular meridians, to communicate among different meridians, and to regulate the flow of Qi and blood along the meridians.

4. Qi is a term used to refer to a type of energy. In Chinese medical theory, it is seen as an essential entity that cannot be seen but is there.

2
Yin/Yang and the Five Elements

To comprehend the history of Chinese medical theory, it is important to understand the central philosophies that underlie medical practice. Unlike Western medicine, in which science gradually replaced philosophy over time as the means to understand and treat disease, in China the practice of medicine has never been separated from its philosophy. Instead, science has taken its place as an important adjunct to, not a replacement for, the philosophical framework of medical theory.

From the beginning, the central goal in Chinese medicine has been to regain and maintain balance, or harmony, among the parts of the body and between the person and his/her environment. A Chinese doctor examines a patient's pulse, tongue, skin tone, behavior, and many other clues as well as physical signs and symptoms to diagnose a problem and suggest a cure; basing his conclusion on the philosophical underpinnings of Chinese medicine that are derived from the two theories of Yin/Yang and Five Elements. Both of these important concepts seem to have been in evidence since long before the earliest writings on medical theory.

Yin/Yang Theory

During the Shang and Zhou Dynasties (c. 1766–249 B.C.), it was fashionable to predict fortunes using various methods.

One of these was "eight Gua," recorded as a tool in one of the oldest books on philosophy, *Yi Jing* (popularized in the West under the older spelling, *I Ching*). The Eight Gua method was based on various combinations of two elements: Qian (≡) and Kun (≡ ≡), represented by groups of three combinations of a solid or broken line. Qian and Kun are meant to symbolize Yin and Yang, the two opposing forces in the universe.

Yin and Yang have no fixed definition, but they are generally taken to represent all the pairs of opposites that express the dualism of the cosmos. Some examples of these opposing aspects are:

Yin	**Yang**
female	male
dark	light
cold	warm
soft	firm
earth	heaven
night	day
empty	full

Yin and Yang, however, must be understood as relational concepts; that is, an object or idea is not absolutely hard or soft, dark or light, per se, but only in comparison to other objects or ideas. Traditional Chinese Medicine applies these relationships to the human body, determining that, for example, the back is relatively Yang and the abdomen is relatively Yin; the outside is relatively Yang and the inside relatively Yin, and so on. The internal organs are also differentiated by Yin and Yang. For example, the six hollow organs (Fu/Bowels) are relatively Yang, the five firm organs (Zang/Viscera) are relatively Yin. Furthermore, there is Yin in Yang, and Yang in Yin. Thus, the heart belongs to Yin relative to the small intestine, but in comparison to the kidneys, it belongs to Yang.

The concept of Yin/Yang dates back before any written history that is available to scholars. The earliest medical textbook, the *Nei Jing* (see chapter 1), which was probably written some time between 200 B.C. and 200 A.D., refers to the Yin/Yang theory as an integral part of the diagnosis and treatment of disease. It states, "The principle of Yin Yang is the basis of everything in creation, the cause of all transformations, and the origin of life and death. . . . If Yin is greater than Yang, Yang will be sick and the person will suffer from cold; if Yang is greater than Yin, Yin will be sick, and the person will suffer fever. Moreover, if Yang is deficient, the outer body will be cold. If Yin is deficient, there will be heat inside the body. If Yang is hyperactive, the outer body will be cold. If Yin is deficient, there will be heat inside the body. If Yang is hyperactive, the outer body will be hot; if Yin is hyperactive, the inner body will be cold inside." *Nei Jing* reinforces this conclusion by saying, "A good doctor will always first observe the color and take the pulse to ascertain Yin Yang." (See chapter 4 for a discussion about diagnosis using pulse points and other indicators.)

In the ideal healthy condition, Yin and Yang are in balance. Imbalance, either of excess or of deficiency, will cause disease. To cure disease, therefore, is to balance the Yin and Yang of the body.

Five Elements Theory

What the essential materials of the universe are, and the truth about their relationship to the human body, have been the subject of inquiry by medical practitioners and theorists all over the globe. In ancient Greece, for instance, Hippocrates and Galen applied Empedocles' four-element theory to human beings and out of this developed their "Doctrine of the Four

Humours," which became the most powerful concept in medieval thinking. At about the same time, Chinese physicians were developing their five-element theory to explain the nature and etiology of disease.

The four elements of the Greek system (fire, water, air, earth) reflected early physicians' beliefs that the human body was a microcosm of the larger universe; according to this theory, the body would be composed of, and be influenced by, the same elements that were apparent in the natural world. Chinese philosopher/physicians identified five elements—water, fire, wood, metal, and earth—and viewed their influence on the body slightly differently.

The five elements are first mentioned in a book called *Shang Shu*, one of the oldest comprehensive philosophical texts known (c. 220 B.C.). This book identified these five elements as the basic and necessary substances of life. There was no mystery about their characteristics and functions.

The interrelationship among the five elements is understood according to certain sequences. For example, when water nourishes grass and trees, making them grow, this is named "water generating wood." Burning wood can catch fire; this is named "wood generating fire." Ashes from the burning wood can produce clay; this is "fire generating earth." Metal is found buried in the earth; this is called "earth generating metal." The melting of the metal to liquid is called "metal generating water." Using the same reasoning, the patterns of restriction may be summarized as follows: water puts out fire, fire melts metal, metal cuts wood, wooden plows turn the earth, and an earthen dam will stop the flow of water.

When the Five Elements theory was incorporated into medical theory, the key was not the elements themselves, but rather the characteristics and interrelationships among them.

Their attributes were extended to everything in the world, including the climates of the four seasons and the human physiological, pathological, and emotional conditions. The following chart summarizes these relationships:

Element	Climate	Season	Physio-logical organ	Emotion	Taste	Color	Ancient Chinese musical tone
Wood	Wind	Spring	Liver	Anger	Sourness	Blue	Jiao
Fire	Heat	Summer	Heart	Joy	Bitterness	Red	Zheng
Earth	Damp	Long-summer	Spleen	Thinking	Sweet	Yellow	Gong
Metal	Dry	Autumn	Lung	Grief	Acridity	White	Shang
Water	Cold	Winter	kidney	Fright	Saltiness	Black	Yu

(Note: "long-summer" is another name for what we call Indian summer, a time of heat and humidity after summer and before autumn. The emotion of "thinking" refers to what we might call anxiety or agitation. The colors in the chart correspond to the patient's complexion when afflicted with a disease associated with a particular organ. This principle is also used when prescribing herbal medicine: a white plant or fruit, for instance, may be used to direct the medicine to alleviate a lung disease.)

Clearly, the emphasis in Chinese medicine was on the functional system, rather than on the structural organ, continuing the holistic viewpoint that has been the basis for Chinese medicine from the beginning. As can be seen from the chart of associated factors above, the patient was evaluated not only in terms of a particular physical affliction or set of symptoms, but also in terms of his or her emotional state, possible influences from the natural environment, and many other considerations. Thus the term "liver" does not mean only the organ; it also represents the functional sphere within the body that corresponds to the season of regeneration, quickening, and fertility.

The ancient theory of Five Elements, as applied to human physiology, simplifies complicated pathology even today. For example, if a patient suffers convulsions or spasms of the calves, these "moving disorders" are recognized as a problem of the liver. The reasoning is as follows: Moving is a property of the wind, and wind is related to the liver. So to treat this disease, the physician must soothe the liver, thereby calming the wind. Similarly, if a patient suffers from abdominal distention, diarrhea, low energy level, and wiry (tight and thready) pulse in the wrist, this indicates a problem related to the spleen. This can be immediately diagnosed as wood overpowering earth, due to the wiry pulse, which is a liver pulse. Calming the liver and encouraging the spleen can cure this problem.

The Connection between Philosophy and Science

Systematic medical theories develop gradually, over time, based on scattered clinical experience and the knowledge gained from primitive observation. Since the natural sciences were relatively undeveloped at the time early medical theory was being formulated, there were no technical tools available for study and verification of theories, such as microscopes and biochemistry techniques. Therefore, ancient doctors simply applied their updated philosophical theories in the medical field. Then, as the natural sciences developed, more and more sophisticated equipment and tools were invented that allowed the philosophical theories to be tested.

This is what occurred in the early nineteenth century, when, with the advent of technology, medieval medicine (as descended from the Greeks and Romans) discarded its philosophic frame and merged with natural science. Because of this rapid growth and expansion of Western medicine, with its many newly effective therapeutic results, many older, philosophically based medical systems declined or were dismissed as irrelevant and outdated.

Traditional Chinese Medicine was faced with that challenge when Western medicine was introduced into China in about 1910. With the establishment of the People's Republic of China, great controversy erupted in China about whether to keep or discard Traditional Chinese Medicine. Western medicine has now been fully integrated and well developed in China. The two healthcare systems—Western and Chinese—complement each other and are now practiced side by side, both in private practice and in hospitals, to the great benefit of patients. It is heartening to witness the successful integration of two systems that seem to be diametrically opposed.

Unlike what occurred with the course of Western medicine, however, Chinese medical theory, perhaps due to its flexibility, harmonized well with the analytical format of Western-style medicine. It is important to note, however, that Traditional Chinese Medicine has never been (and under no circumstances should be) separated from its early philosophical theories, such as the five elements and Yin/Yang. These basic philosophical concepts were deeply implanted in Chinese medicine from the beginning, penetrating basic pathological, pharmacological, and diagnostic beliefs. These two important theories have, of course, developed over the years to encompass a much larger application than their original context, and they have proved themselves remarkably resilient. Modern diagnostic methods and treatments still are based on these fundamental philosophical theories.

3
Influences of the Three Great Philosophies

Three great philosophies have influenced China: Daoism, Confucianism, and Buddhism. All of these also had some influence on the development of Chinese medicine.

Daoism

The true origins of Daoism are lost in history, but it appears along with Confucianism as a major philosophical movement in the latter part of the Chou Dynasty (1122–249 B.C.). Daoism did not develop into an organized religion until the early centuries of the Christian era.

The founder of Daoism, and the author to which one of the major texts of this philosophy, the *Dao de Jing*, is attributed, is the great sage Lao Zi. According to legend, Lao Zi was incredibly long-lived, and one day after many years simply started walking west, across the border of China into the great wastes of what is now known as Siberia, and was never seen again.

The word "Dao" means simply "way." The "way" in Daoism, unlike the same word used in Confucianism (see below), has a metaphysical meaning, referring to a nameless, formless, eternal principle that rests behind everything in the universe. The original followers of Daoism were probably hermits or recluses, seeking the meaning of life in contemplation of the Dao.

The early Daoists believed that life is the greatest possession, and they often practiced asceticisms in order to prolong life as well as to gain mystical insight. Later practitioners, beginning in the later Han Dynasty (3rd century A.D.), began to transform what had begun as a pure philosophy into occultism and alchemy. From these experiments eventually arose a series of charlatans and magicians who concerned themselves chiefly with the writing of charms, the expelling of devils, and other superstitious practices.

Ironically, perhaps, Daoism contributed to the development of medicine chiefly because of this alchemical inquiry. In their search for the perfect elixirs, which could prolong life and beauty, they experimented with and recorded the effects of many herbs and minerals. The results of their experiments helped to develop pharmaceutical technique and contributed to the development of medicines used for surgical diseases and wound healing, and their documentation is a great help in the study of ancient chemistry and pharmaceutics.

A second way in which Daoism contributed to Chinese medicine is in the development of the art of deep breathing. The beneficial effects of breath control on health are stated in the *Dao de Jing* and were further developed by Zhuang Zi (230–220 B.C.) and Ge Hong of the Jin Dynasty (265–416 A.D.). In the prescribed method of breathing, the person strives to breathe so as not to hear the sound of inhalation or exhalation. The rule is to inhale generously and exhale sparingly. One prescribed test is to suspend a feather of the wild goose in front of the nose and mouth and try not to have the feather stir while the breath is being expelled. With gradual practice, one would increase the count of heartbeats during which the breath is held. After a very long period of time, it was believed, one should be able to count a thousand heartbeats. When an old man has arrived at that stage, he will be transformed into a young man, each day adding to the transformation. These breathing exercises were probably the origin of the breathing techniques later found in the practice of Qi Gong (see chapter 7).

Buddhism

Introduced into China from India by the 1st century A.D. (some say up to two centuries earlier), Buddhism taught the suppression of passions and the cultivation of such qualities as charity, compassion, harmlessness, and poverty. The Buddhists believe that life and the world are illusory, and that peace of mind comes from emptying one's mind in meditation.

In China, Buddhism began as a practice of foreigners, but gradually gained favor among the Chinese, largely because of its doctrine of escape from the suffering and burdens of life. Under the later rulers of the Tang Dynasty (618–906 A.D.), Buddhism was officially approved and gained more and more Chinese followers.

Buddhism's major contribution to Chinese medicine lies in its practice of the art of meditation, achieved through a system of gradual relaxation and repose. This practice was considered the gateway to health and also believed to contribute to immortality. Eventually it was incorporated into the Qi Gong, which is still taught and practiced in China. Many well-known doctors were either Buddhists or Daoists.

Confucianism

Confucius was a great ethical teacher who lived in about the 4th century B.C. We know of him primarily through a book written by his disciples some two generations after his death, called *The Analects of Confucius*. Recognized as a great teacher during his lifetime, he was so revered in later centuries that he has sometimes appeared godlike, and his ethical teachings evolved into religious rituals followed by millions of Chinese.

Confucius seems to have concerned himself less with metaphysics than with those principles that contribute to the stability, peace, and prosperity of society, the family, and the individual. His teachings emphasize that there is a divine order to the universe that works for love and righteousness, and prescribes how a person should act in order to be in harmony with that universe and find his or her higher good.

Like Daoism, Confucianism refers to the "way," or "Dao," but in Confucianism, the Way refers not to the metaphysical way of the Daoists, but to a practical, moral principle embodied in the rites and attitudes of ethical behavior.

It was this ethical emphasis in Confucianism that greatly influenced Chinese physicians, whose reverence for life and self-prescribed duty to help those in need echoed the humanistic Confucian doctrine.

II
Diagnosis and Treatment

4

Like Wood Floating on Water: Diagnosis Techniques in Chinese Medicine

Traditional Chinese Medicine is unique in the methods used to diagnose illness. Whereas in Western medicine the doctor relies primarily on the patient's reported symptoms and the results of laboratory tests (what in Chinese medical theory would be referred to as diagnosis "away from the body"), in Chinese medicine the doctor uses a combination of techniques to observe the whole person. There are four main classes of inquiry: 1) observation of the patient's tongue, complexion, eyes, and manner; 2) palpation, namely, the intensity, speed, and rhythm of the pulse; 3) listening and smelling; and 4) questioning the patient about such things as heat and cold, thirst, hearing, elimination, sleep, menstruation, and so on. Beginning medical students are taught an ancient poem that reminds them of these four essential components to diagnosis.

Pulse Diagnosis

This is the technique: The doctor puts his index, middle, and ring fingers of either hand on the ulnar artery in the wrist of the patient.[1] From the intensity, speed, and rhythm of the pulse, he can determine the state of all internal organs. For example, a "floating" pulse indicates exterior syndrome: cold or flu, allergic reaction. A "wiry" pulse indicates pain and liver Qi stagnation. Traditionally, different portions of the left and right pulse are attributed to the organs of the respective sides. The right wrist, from wrist to elbow, reflects the lung, spleen/stomach, and right kidney (also called the "life gate"). The left wrist reflects the heart, liver, and left kidney. Both wrists, then, must be examined by the doctor for a complete diagnosis.[2] There are six principal pulses and many variations. The pulse varies as the disease progresses (allowing the doctor to use the pulse in prognosis as well as diagnosis), and also varies according to the season. All these variables make pulse diagnosis an exacting and complicated science.

No one knows exactly how the pulse diagnosis technique evolved, because there is no extant text that introduces the technique; one of the earliest known medical texts—the *Nei Jing* (500 B.C.–200 A.D.)—refers to an *updated* form of the procedure. According to the *Nei Jing*, the procedure in use up to that time required the doctor to check three separate pulse positions of the body (neck, wrist, and foot) in order to make an accurate diagnosis. *Nei Jing* stated definitively that taking the pulse at the wrist alone is acceptable for making the correct diagnosis.

The pulse diagnosis technique was refined during the earliest centuries of medical development. Besides the *Nei Jing*, descriptions of the technique appear in another important text called *Nan Jing*, (206 B.C.–220 A.D.) as well as in the writings of many notable physicians such as Bian Que, Chun Yu Yi, Po Wong, and Zhang Zhong Jing (Bian Que, Chun Yu Yi, and Po Wong are described later in this chapter; that of Zhang Zhong Zing is described in chapter 1).

During the Jin Dynasty (265–420 A.D.), a doctor named Wang Shu He wrote an entire text on pulse diagnosis—which he called *Mai Jing*—after amassing the existing data on the subject and performing his own experiments. This then was the first specialized research documented in Chinese medical history. Wang Shu He also served the government as administrator of the Royal Institute of Health.

He stated in the preface to *Mai Jing*, "Pulse diagnosis is a very difficult and delicate technique. It is difficult to distinguish between the pulses in concept and the actual clinical reading of them. Deep (chen) can be mistaken for hiding (fu) and the subsequent treatment will be wrong. Similarly, if the soft (huan) pulse is wrongly identified as the slow (chi) pulse, the normal treatment will be dangerous." In clinical practice, it is common to encounter patients who have multiple problems, making pulse diagnosis difficult. Also, different cases may evidence the same pulse pattern. For instance, the "tight" and "wiry" pulses may be confused, or the "rapid" and "forceful," or the "feeble" and "weak."

Wang Shu He, who has been called the "Father of Pulse Diagnosis," defined Cun Kou, wrist-position pulse-taking, and definitively linked the pulse in the three portions of the wrist to specific organs in the body (see footnote 1 of this chapter). He thus resolved the key problem in pulse diagnosis—how to use pulse diagnosis to ascertain the condition of the major organs—and promoted the wrist pulse-taking technique to its now-popular standing. All subsequent pulse-diagnosis theories have been based on his writings. Wang Shu He classified pulse patterns into twenty-four variants and also compared similar pulses, describing how to distinguish one pulse from another.

Wang Shu's next step was to make the connection between pulse diagnosis and treatment. He wrote, for example, "A stroke and headache patient often has a tight (jin) pulse," and "a patient with arteriosclerosis always has a tight pulse." He further stated, "Hiding (fu) pulse indicates cholera due to severe dehydration. The effective circulatory blood volume is not sufficient for finding the pulse easily; one must exert great pressure to detect it."

Regarding malaria, he also had valuable insight: "A malaria patient has a wiry (xian) pulse. If this appears together with a rapid (shu) pulse, there is heat inside. Wiry (xian) and slow (chi) together means cold inside, and weak pulse signifies deficiency; irregular (dai) and scattered (san) pulses indicate a dangerous situation." His diagnosis of lung abscess also involved an ingenious observation: "A slight pain in the chest lung area, accompanied by a rolling and rapid pulse, indicates a lung abscess. This should be treated with platycodon root decoction." (This treatment is used successfully to this day.)

During the Five Dynasties era (907–960 A.D.), Dr. Gao Yang Sheng wrote a book called *Wang Shu He Mai Jue* ("Wang Shu He's Precious Poem for Pulse Diagnosis"), crediting the father of pulse diagnosis in the title. Gao's book was organized in the form of poems, which made it easier for doctors to understand, recite, and remember the principles of pulse diagnosis, thus popularizing the system even further.

A doctor who excelled at diagnosis: Guo Yu.

During the East Han Dynasty (202 B.C.–220 A.D.), in Si Chuan Province, there lived an old fisherman known in history as Po Wong (his real name is unknown). His medical technique was said to be excellent, and he wrote two books, one on acupuncture and the other on pulse diagnosis (both have been lost). His techniques were passed down, however, to his apprentice and to that person's apprentice, who also became a well-known doctor. His name was Guo Yu, and Guo Yu also lived in Si Chuan Province, circa 50–130 A.D. His specialties, like his predecessor's, were pulse diagnosis and acupuncture.

During the East Han Dynasty, Guo Yu served the King of He as the chief doctor for the emperor and royal family. As a test, the king had a man and a woman lie side by side hidden under a mosquito net. Each one stretched out one wrist for Guo Yu to check. Yu said, "The pulse is a man's, the right is a woman's. How can one have a mixed pulse?" The king was amazed and delighted by Guo Yu's obvious expertise.

The first published case studies were those of a doctor named Chun Yu Yi, a notable physician of the Han Dynasty who was once imprisoned for refusing to treat some corrupt officials. He was released when his daughter interceded for him in a letter to the emperor, who, apparently intrigued by Chun Yu Yi's medical knowledge and scruples, interviewed him in detail about his expertise and method of training his students. Chun Yu Yi subsequently was able to work for the government while maintaining his private practice.

Chun Yu Yi outlined twenty-five case histories in his book *Zhen Ji,* in which he gave for each patient the name, sex, occupation, address, pathology, diagnosis, treatment, and prognosis. His original notes are lost, but they were recorded for posterity by Sima Qian in the *Shi Ji,* where they earned distinction as the first published case studies.

Chun Yu Yi specialized in diagnosis by observation. For example, upon seeing one of the servants of the court premier, he remarked, "Look at his complexion; there is a sign of disease." Although the patient did not feel sick, Chun pointed out that by a simple glance he could detect a sallow, dark-yellow tone; further checking revealed a dull, bluish tinge. He predicted, "This is a case of spleen damage; in spring, the patient will feel obstruction and experience difficulty in swallowing. By summer, the patient will die of stool bleeding." The prognosis proved to be entirely accurate.

In addition to emphasizing observation, Chun Yu Yi also contributed to the development of diagnosis through pulse monitoring. Among the twenty-five previously mentioned case studies, ten patients were evaluated and prognosticated using this method. Many pulse patterns already had been described in the book *Nei Jing.* In Chun Yu Yi's *Zhen Ji,* more than twenty of these were discussed, such as floating (fu), deep (chen), slow (chi), rapid (shu), rolling (hua), hesitant (se), long (chang), big (da), small (xiao), irregular (dai), and wiry (Xian). Except for some of the additional pulses mentioned—firm (jian), flat (ping), drum (gu), quiet (jing), and restless (zao)—most of these pulse patterns have been continuously recognized in clinical practice ever since.

Chun Yu Yi's treatment methods included herbal medicine, acupuncture, moxibustion, and ice application. He is also credited with the inventions of gargling with herbal preparations. During the Western Han Dynasty, it was considered efficacious, after having taken a medicine for longevity, to swallow a preparation made of stones. On learning this, Chun Yu Yi immediately warned people of the danger of this practice.

Regarding medicine during the Song and Yuan dynastic period in China (960–1368 A.D.), the extant texts summarize diagnostic experiences and documents. Doctor Cui Jia Yan wrote a book based on the earlier *Nan Jing,* in which, addressing the floating, deep, slow, and rapid pulses as main topics, he correlated the twenty-four pulses more exactly to their pathogenic factors, such as wind, Qi (energy), cold, and heat. This made the pulse diagnostic technique more accurate. Of special note is that Cui was the first author to record the pulse types Lao and Ge (Lao pulse is deep and slow, with no flexibility; Ge pulse feels like a leather strip; both indicate a fatal condition). As a mnemonic device, the book was written in the form of a poem. This book remained popular in subsequent generations and was reedited several times by later doctors.

In 1241, Shi Fa wrote a book on pulse diagnosis, which he illustrated with thirty-three charts. He used a new method of classification for the twenty-four pulses: Qi Biao, Ba Li, and Jiu Dao. Qi Biao means "seven exteriors," Ba Li, "eight interiors," and Jiu Dao, the "nine channels." How to make a prognosis based on the pulse taking was discussed in detail. Shi Fa's book also includes the first mention of other diagnostic factors in practice at the time, such as to listen, to observe, and to check for odors.

During the next century, two additional works on pulse diagnosis appeared; the later work included chapters on using the existing pulse diagnostic techniques for conditions occurring within the specialties of gynecology and pediatrics.

Observation of the Tongue As a Diagnostic Technique

Diagnosis by Chinese medical doctors also commonly includes observation of the tongue. The beginnings of the use of this method also are unknown, although it is mentioned in several of the earliest medical texts such as *Shang Han Lun*, written by the renowned doctor Zhang Zhong Jing (see chapter 1). The first doctor to devote an entire text to this subject was Du Ben, who lived during the Yuan Dynasty (1260–1368). Du Ben enhanced his book with thirty-six colored charts to show the various shades of color of the tongue and its coatings, and to illustrate the various properties of the body of the tongue. Three main tongue colors were recorded: pale, red, and blue. The surface was described as having a red sting, red star, cracks, and other patterns. Colors of the coating included white, yellow, gray, and black, while its quality could be dry, slippery, coarse, prickly, uneven, and splitting. These various tongue signs were correlated with specific syndromes, including comments on pathology, etiology, and prognosis.

Pulse and tongue diagnosis both had been well developed before the Ming and Qing Dynasties (1368–1912). During the Ming-Qing period, no new diagnostic techniques were developed. The significant contribution made in diagnostic technique during this period was the correction of diagnostic prejudice (which emphasized pulse diagnosis alone) and the emphasis on combining diagnostic tools to get a more comprehensive view. The four diagnostic techniques are observation (complexion, tongue, stool, urine), smell, inquiry, and palpation (pulse, abdomen). Each offers a unique view of the condition of the body, and by using all of them, it was believed, a doctor could avoid being misled by false symptoms.

In 1723, Doctor Lin Zhi Han wrote a book that reflected this viewpoint. To emphasize the importance of inquiry diagnosis, Li Yan listed fifty-five items that should be inquired about before making a diagnosis. Another doctor of this period, Zhang Jie Bin, wrote a poem to facilitate remembering all the points of inquiry. It reads as follows: "First ask the patient's temperature sensation, second is sweating or not and how, third about head and body, fourth about bowel movement, and urination, fifth is about diet, sixth is about chest, seventh is about hearing ability, eighth is about thirst or lack, ninth is about smelling sensation, and tenth is about mind condition—clear or confused." This is still considered a useful guide for a young doctor inquiring about the patient's condition.

A Physician Who Excelled at Diagnosis: Bian Que.

The first Chinese physician whose biography was officially recorded in history books is the great Bian Que. Excerpts from Bian Que's writings were recorded in several classical history books. He lived circa 500 B.C. in He Bei Province. As a young man, he was working as a manager in a hotel when he met a guest named Chang San Jun, who was an expert in medical techniques. Intrigued by the man's skill and knowledge, Bian Que followed him to study medicine and, after finishing his training, practiced medicine in several counties. He wrote two books, but both have been lost over time. Bian Que excelled in the diagnostic techniques of olfaction, inquiry, and palpation, and was especially famous for his observation and pulse-taking. Acknowledgement of his special talent appears in Zhang Zhong Jing's treatise several hundred years later.

Some examples of Bian Que's proficiency are included in his biography. Once, for example, Bian Que observed the complexion of the King of Qi Huan, detected disease, and informed the monarch that he needed immediate treatment. After ignoring this and several subsequent warnings, the king succumbed to his disease. A story concerning Bian Que's utilization of the pulse diagnosis technique is even more fascinating. He was summoned to treat the prince of Zhao state, who had been unconscious for five days. After taking the prince's pulse, Bian Que advised, "His pulse is normal; there is nothing to be concerned about." A few days later, the prince completely recovered. On another occasion, Bian Que was passing through Guo state (around Henan and Shan Xi) and heard that the prince of Guo had suddenly died of some disease. Bian Que consulted with the royal physician, asking for more information. Bian Que's diagnosis was that the prince was suffering from false death syndrome (Shi Jue or shock). Bian Que directed his student, Zhi Yang, to administer acupuncture, and the prince regained consciousness. He then directed another student, Bao, to administer two different medicinal formulas to warm the prince's hypochondriac (upper abdominal) area. Following this treatment, the prince was able to sit up, and after twenty days of oral medication, he experienced a complete recovery.

Bian Que excelled in internal medicine, surgery, ophthalmology, gynecology, pediatrics, and ear, nose, and throat medicine. It is said that a man named Li Xi, the premier of the province of Qin, was jealous of Bian Que's superior medical knowledge and sent assassins to kill him as he was traveling through the province. Although another well-known doctor of his generation had been murdered by the jealous official, Bian Que escaped. After his death he was memorialized by the Chinese people, and many of his relics were preserved in Henan and Shan Xi.

Notes

1. According to the ancient medical text *Nan Jing*, the pulse extends for one and nine-tenths of an inch along the wrist. This space is divided into

three parts, called "inch," "bar," and "cubit," each of which has its particular pulse variation.

2. The various pulsations are described quite precisely in the texts as having particular characteristics. For instance, a "deep" pulse is said to be like a stone thrown into water. A "superficial" pulse is like a piece of wood floating on water.

5

A Thousand Golden Formulas: The Development of Herbal Medicine

Shen Nong was the second of the legendary "celestial emperors," who supposedly resigned from 2838 B.C. to 2698 B.C. He is credited with the discovery of and experimentation with medicinal herbs—a significant attribution considering the continuing importance of herbs in Chinese medicine. Shen Nong, blessed with a "transparent stomach," purportedly took as many as seventy different medicinal plants in one day, including extremely toxic preparations for which he was then able to devise antidotes. His contributions were memorialized in the first treatise on Chinese herbal medicine, from which many of the principles of Chinese pharmacology were established or clearly defined for the first time. This book is called *Shen Nong Ben Cao Jing*. The words "ben cao" translate as "botanical medicine," so the title of this work becomes "Shen Nong's book on botanical medicine," or "Shen Nong's Pharmacopoeia."

Although credited to the celestial emperor, likely as a measure of respect, this book was probably compiled much later—sometime between 200 B.C. and 200 A.D.—by a number of prominent physicians, as is the case with many other ancient Chinese scientific texts. In China there is a feeling that one's ancestors and predecessors are to be respected and consulted, and most medical texts begin with extensive research into the work of the author's forebears.

Shen Nong Ben Cao Jing is composed of three volumes and lists 365 medicines. Of these, 252 are described as being derived form botanical sources, sixty-seven from animal sources, and forty-six from mineral sources. These 365 medicines were further categorized according to their properties and function. Belonging to the "upper" category are 120 medicines, defined as generally having little or no toxicity, and which can be used as tonic and preventive medicines for health and longevity. The "medium" category also includes 120 medicines; of these, some are nontoxic, but most have a tonic function as well as a function for curing disease. The third "lower," category includes 125 medicines. These are established as adjuncts and messengers[1] in medicinal formulas "for treating disease responding to earth" (meaning caused by environmental factors). Most of the medicines in this category are toxic, thus rendering them fit only for temporary use.

Besides simply listing medicines, the *Shen Nong Pharmacopoeia* also set forth some basic principles of pharmacology having to do with classification, theory, and application that are still used today by Chinese pharmacists and physicians.

1. Medicinal substances were divided into four categories by property (cold, hot, warm, and cool) and five flavors (sour, bitter, acrid, salty, and sweet). A uniform classification system made the identification and use of herbal substances much easier for physicians.

2. The pharmacopoeia stated the principles that should be followed when combining herbs and described the roles played by individual herbs such as Jun (chief), Chen (assistant), Zuo (adjunct), and Shi (messenger). In a particular formula, only one ingredient will be the "chief" or curing ingredient; it is combined with other substances to help it achieve its intended effect.

3. The theory of interaction recognized that not all medicines can be combined successfully; on the other hand, some

may enhance the effects of others. In other words, some combinations of herbs increase therapeutic effect; others can reduce the therapeutic effect; others can aid reduction of side effects; and still others can cause severe side effects.

4. The pharmacopoeia emphasized the importance of collection times, pharmaceutical techniques, and procedures. Before the herbs were taken as medicine, it was always necessary to prepare the herbs according to specific pharmaceutical principles in order for their medicinal properties to be available. (For more on preparation techniques, see p. 59.)

5. More than 170 specific diseases were named as being treatable by the 365 listed medicines. The list includes internal diseases, gynecological problems, five diseases of the sensory organs, and conditions requiring surgery. Most functions of the medicines described in this seminal book have since been verified as accurate by modern science, and many of these cures are still used in clinical practice. For example, ephedra is still used to treat asthma, dichroa (Chang Shan) is effective for malaria, coptis root is used for dysentery, seaweed for thyroid goiter, polyporos as a diuretic, and scutelliaria root for pneumonia.

Shen Nong's Pharmacopoeia is still studied by students of Traditional Chinese Medicine as a valuable reference work.

Other, even older, texts from this earliest period in Chinese medicine show that the experimental tradition of the celestial emperor was carried on by later physicians as they continued to identify and classify new medicines and connect them with particular diseases. A book surviving from the Zhou Dynasty called *Zhou Li* (written c. 550–221 B.C.) states: "five odors, five grains, and five medicines were used to help the patient recover; five Qi [odors], five tones, and five colors can be used for prognosis," and "for skin problems [Yang], stop their progress with five toxins, nourish with five Qi, treat with five medicines." As used in this text, "five medicines" does not refer to specific drugs, but rather to specific classifications of that time.[2]

Shi Jing, one of the extant documents from the West Zhou Dynasty (1122–771 B.C.), contains a historical reference to medicines used in the earlier Shang Dynasty (c. 1766–1122 B.C.). *Shi Jing* mentions more than fifty botanicals used medically, including plantago seed, alisma tuber, pueraria root, swallow-wort, sweet wormwood, licorice root, scutellaria root, and fritillary bulb. The book also recommends the best times and methods for collection and the best sources for these herbs—the earliest reference to how herbs should be collected and stored.

A later text, *Shan Hai Jing*, is the oldest geography text of the Qin Dynasty (221–207 B.C.). It is included in this discussion on herbal medicine because, in addition to other geographical matters, the book recorded clearly the areas of production, properties, functions and indications of over 120 medicines from animal, botanical, mineral, and even aquatic origin. More than ten diseases—covering internal, gynecological, ophthalmic, and dermatologic conditions—are mentioned as being treatable by the medicines in *Shan Hai Jing*. Many of the medicines are mentioned as having tonic and preventive functions as well as curative uses. This information is valuable in tracing how preventive medicine evolved. As we will see, prevention is one of the central goals of Traditional Chinese Medicine, and these early texts show that this standard was in practice over two thousand years ago.

In this book, we notice the first mention of how to administer the herbal medicines. Both oral and external administration of the medicines were described; external methods included bathing in, lying on, and applying the medicine via a patch (probably the earliest use of this type of medication delivery). Patches are a common way of administering certain medicines today: for example, a popular formula called Shang Shi Zhi

Teng Gao is administered via patch for arthritis caused by joints injured by a damp and humid environment. The patch helps the body eliminate the dampness and also relieves pain. The *Shan Hai Jing* also stated that some reaction to medicine is normal. For example, it was written, "if there is no dizziness or slight vertigo, there will be no cure."

The *Nei Jing* is a another important text in Chinese medicine that dates from at least 250 B.C. Its text alludes to more than twenty earlier medical textbooks that have since been lost, and, like *Shen Nong Ben Cao Jing*, it seems to have been compiled by many physicians over many years. This book is significant in the development of Chinese medicine because it is the first time a medical text discusses herbal formulas, or combinations of medicines, as opposed to single applications. It records thirteen medicinal formulas as treatment for manic syndrome, women's menstrual problems, and other types of diseases.

A great deal of progress in the art of herbal medicine occurred during the next several hundred years, especially during the Tang Dynasty (618–906), whose government encouraged the development of the medical arts in many ways, including the development of a national pharmacopoeia. During this period, many privately published pharmacopoeias appeared as well. The many extant texts help us clearly trace the progress of medicinal and pharmacological theories. Some of the most important are described below:

Ben Jing Ji Zhu

During the several hundred years since the compilation of *Shen Nong Ben Cao Jing* (see above), many new medicines had been discovered and new experiences were recorded as physicians carried on the experimental methods of the legendary celestial emperor in order to confirm the properties and functions of some herbal medicines and to make modifications to earlier ideas about others.

Ben Jing Ji Zhu was written by Tao Hong Jing (452–536 A.D.). As a young man, Tao Hong Jing became involved in Daoist activities, which affected him so deeply that he adopted the religion. A prolific medical writer, his understanding of the theories of Yin and Yang, and the Five Elements, was unsurpassed.

To the 365 herbal medicines recorded in *Sheng Nog Ben Cao Jing*, Tao Hong Jing added another 365, which he selected from three important medical texts of the period. While *Shen Nong Ben Cao Jing* had classified the medicines according to upper, medium, and lower properties, Tao Hong Jing changed that classification to seven categories: Jade and Stone, Grass, Wood, Animal Product, Fruit and Vegetable, Rice and Food, and You Ming Wu Yong ("named without function," meaning those medicines whose particular applications were not known). With regard to the properties of medicine, he pointed out that the distinction between the cold and hot properties of medicine should be clearly made, and he assigned each medicine to one of eight levels: cold, slightly cold, very cold, neutral, warm, slightly warm, very warm, and hot. His book also contains a list of the most commonly used herbal medicines of his time.

Xin Xiu Ben Cao

Around 657 A.D., a physician named Su Jing proposed to the Tang government that a reedited pharmacopoeia was needed. The project was approved, and two years later, the work of Su Jing and that of twenty assistants was published as the first national pharmacopoeia, *Xin Xiu Ben Cao*.

Xin Xiu Ben Cao described 844 various herbal medicines (114 more than in *Ben Jing Ji Zhu*) and added medicinal charts and graphs.

During the editing period, the government ordered the collection of the best local herbs from all parts of the country and hired artists to paint and record them. Medicines from foreign countries (namely, Thailand and Malaysia) were recorded as well, among them curcuma root and benzoin. Many of these are in common use today. This pharmacopoeia corrected many previous mistakes and was respected for a long time as a necessary textbook for reference by doctors.

Privately Published Pharmacopoeias during the Tang Dynasty

Ben Cao Shi Yi replaced the selections on herbal medicine missing from *Xin Xiu Ben Cao*. The author, a Dr. Chen, whose first name is unknown, was apparently a very knowledgeable person who had read many medical books and excelled in botanical classification. He created the "Shi Ji," a ten-principle theory explaining how and why certain medications work. For example, he wrote, "Pungent medicine (ginger root, bitter orange peel) can be used to disperse an obstruction. Herbs with dry properties (mulberry bark and phaseolous seed) can remove dampness/humidity." This theory became very popular and is still the fundamental principle for the creation of Chinese medicinal formulas.

Yue Wang Ben Cao, written by the Tibetan doctor Ma Ya Na and others, recorded 329 medicines. Much philosophy and pathology, as well as some special catheterization methods, were also included. *Hai Yao Ben Cao,* written by Li Xun, whose family originally came from Arabia, is a collection of information on 124 foreign fragrance medications.

Shi Liao Ben Cao, a summary of medicinal foods, was written by Meng She during the Tang Dynasty. Its special contribution was establishing foodstuffs as a medicinal source. This subject was further elaborated on by Shi Liang Chen (934 A.D.) who wrote *Shi Xing Ben Cao,* in which he further developed the field of medicinal foodstuffs introduced by Meng She and emphasized the importance of the properties of food.

"A Tang Dynasty Physician"

Sun Si Mao was an important physician of the Tang Dynasty who lived between 581 and 682 A.D. and made many contributions to Chinese medicine. He studied many baffling diseases of the time and accurately attributed them to diet. Thyroid goiter, for example, he related to the water drunk by people in mountain areas. He also treated night blindness with animal liver. Today, of course, we know that the Vitamin A contained in the liver is beneficial in such cases.

In pharmacology, Sun Si Mao advocated comprehensive therapy, combining herbal medicine with acupuncture, massage, and moxibustion. Prescriptions, he believed, should depend on the differentiation of syndrome. For example, for Xu Lao (deficiency and fatigue) syndrome, he established twenty-five different modes for prescribing the therapeutic formula according to varying cases and constitutions. He was against the abuse of medication, advocating instead that people should collect and store them until needed, recognizing that a store of quality herbs is essential to effect good therapeutic results.

To preserve health, Sun Si Mao advocated managing stress to create a strong foundation for the body, thus maintaining defense against disease and encouraging a long and healthy life. With regard to a healthful diet, he suggested that people should eat regular balanced meals of cooked foods chosen from the five tastes (sour, sweet, acrid, bitter, and salty). After eating, he suggested rinsing the mouth and taking a short, relaxing walk. Thus we may add the precursor of modern gerontology to Sun Si Mao's other contributions!

In acknowledging Sun Si Mao's contributions to medicine, the people called him the "King of Medicine" and built many temples as memorials to him.

Achievements in Pharmaceutical Preparation

Pre-preparation is of paramount importance in achieving the desired effect from medicinal herbs. In the Chinese language, this procedure is called "Pao Zhi." Some basic methods for preparing medicine were described in *Shang Han Lun* (Zhang Zhong Jing's landmark book on medicinal formulas from the second century), such as peeling the cinnamon twig, removing the core from peony bark, and marinating rhubarb root in wine. By following these procedures, the raw material would become medicine, existing properties could be changed, medical effects heightened, side effects reduced, and easy storability attained. During the fifth century A.D., experiences and achievements in this field were summarized in the *Pao Zhi Lun* ("Techniques for Preparing Medicines") by Lei Xiao, a work in which three hundred herbal medicines were described, focusing on property and preparation procedures. Lei Xiao wrote, for example, that croton seed "needs to be broken, fried in vegetable oil or cooked in wine, and ground into a paste before it can be used as medicine." Modern research has borne this out. Toxic oils and protein render the croton seed poisonous; after frying, during which the oil is released and evaporated, the protein is broken down and the seed detoxified. These methods are still used today by Chinese pharmacists.

Lei Xiao categorized pharmaceutical preparation for fourteen methods, including baking, warm dehydration, frying, and water flowing. His book established the basic framework for these techniques.

A National Commission on Pharmacology

During the Song, Jin, and Yuan Dynasties (960–1368 A.D.), special organizations for regulating pharmacology were established. They were charged with storing medicine for the emperor's use, as well as regulating distribution in the medical marketplace.

When Wang An Shi (1010–1085) inaugurated the New Law Period, which provided a beneficient atmosphere for agricultural and economic development in China, herbal medicine was controlled by the government, which held all patents, not trusting the private sector to regulate itself. In 1076, a National Pharmacy was opened by the National Health Administration. From the outset, the National Commission on Pharmacology played a positive role in advocating quality health care. Patented herbal medicine was dispensed in standard doses (which, incidentally, are still used in clinical practice in Traditional Chinese Medicine). In addition, quality control and emergency services were instituted. As time passed, and the government became corrupt later in the Song Dynasty (twelfth and thirteenth centuries) the quality of this agency declined.

In 973 A.D., historical accounts tell us that the Song government assigned nine people, including Liu Han, Ma Zhi, and other officials from the National Health Administration to reedit the national pharmacopoeia. Using three former classics as their main reference sources, and with the addition of 139 new herbal medicines, the new national pharmacopoeia was published with the title *Kai Bao Ben Cao*. Using a new method of categorization, 983 medications were recorded. This new edition influenced herbal medicine until 1057, when it was reedited by two physicians. The new edition described a total of 1,082 herbal medications.

In 1058, the Song government issued an order for the collection of medicinal plants. Specimens (actual or illustrations) had to be noted along with their botanical characteristics, such as climatic requirements, growth cycle, and the best time for harvest. For all important medicines, customs officials and merchants were required to stamp the package with an indication of the original source and submit a sample to the government. More than 150 states were involved in the project. The huge amount of collected information was culled by Su Song in 1061, resulting in the first book that included charts of medicinal plants: *Tu Jing Ben Cao* ("Illustrated Pharmacopoeia"). Consisting of twenty volumes, it recorded data on 780 plants, and charts illustrated 625 medicines.

A milestone in pharmacology was written by Tang Shen Wei (1056–1093) called *Jing Shi Zheng Lei Bei Ji Ben Cao,* commonly called *Zheng Lei Ben Cao.* It listed 1,558 herbal medicines, including more than 476 new ones, and each listing was accompanied by graphic charts and directions for pharmaceutical preparation. Tang's greatest contribution in this text was his explanation and verification of the "channel entered" of each herbal medicine in pharmacologic theory. It also included 3,000 proven formulas and 1,000 explanations for why each component was used.

Zheng Lei Ben Cao became the basis of a new national pharmacopeia when, in 1108, Emperor Zhao Ji (Hui Zong) ordered its reediting by his chief medical officer. In 1249, when another reediting was done by the then-current medical officer, the national pharmacopoeia listed 1,746 herbal medicines.

Several privately published pharmacopoeias during this period expanded on the official work. One of these was *Ben Cao Yan Yi,* written by Kou Zong Bi in 1116 A.D. Listing 460 popular medicines, one of its important contributions was that of quality comparison between the medicines. Because of his abundant experience, research, and observation, the author was able to offer practical advice on how the different medicines worked.

Bao Qing Ben Cao Zhe Zhong was written by Chen Yan, a famed doctor of medicine who had been born in Zhe Jiang Province. His book categorized 789 medications according to their properties and functions. This method of classification is still used in Chinese pharmacopoeias and medical textbooks.

Many innovations in pharmacological theory appear in the writings of doctors in the Jin and Yuan Dynasties (1115–1368 A.D.). *Zhen Zhu Nang* ("Pearl Bag") by Zhang Yuan Su was the most significant pharmacology text during this period. Only a hundred herbal medicines were discussed, but more importantly, the book discussed the development of pharmacological theory and the various properties of the different medications such as flavor, Yin-Yang, Hou Bo (heavy and light), ascending and descending, floating and sinking, tonifying and reducing, and the channel entered.

Tai Ping Hui Min He Ji Ju Fang (1107) updated the procedures for preparation of herbs discussed by Li Xiao in the fifth century (see p. 59). The procedures were augmented to include water preparation, grinding, frying in vinegar or oil, dry frying, baking in paper or flour, roasting over charcoal, marinating, steaming, and other treatments. According to this book, vinegar or wine frying, as well as steaming in wine, made the subsequent medicine work more rapidly and achieve better results. Also, it was reported, herbs baked in wine could improve blood circulation; baking them in vinegar increased their astringent ability. This indicated that Pao Zhi techniques were useful not only for inhibiting side effects of herbal medicines, but also in improving the effectiveness of the medicines.

"The First Steroid"

Records that describe how to produce the medicine Qiu Shi appear in at least two pharmacopoeias of the period (581–682). This technique included two methods, one of which successfully utilized the steroid precipitative reaction (crystallization) with saponin, the earliest pharmaceutical manufacture of a steroid by extraction from urine. With the appearance of these new theories, the pill form also changed: the flour-based pill and liquid forms were created, whereas before the herbs had been simply ground and used in powder form or pressed into rough pills. Coating techniques for pills and tablets were developed during this period, and there was progress as well in overcoming the odor of medicine. For example, one author wrote, "Magnolia bark oil has a bitter taste, which stings the throat and tongue unless marinated in ginger root."

The Role of Diet

The adage "food is medicine" had always been a part of Chinese culture. As we have seen, one of the earliest mentions of the importance of eating properly to maintain health was in the writings of the great physician Sun Si Mao (see p. 78). During the Song and Yuan periods, the proverb took on greater shades of meaning due to the advances brought about by medical research. Special porridges and soups were recommended in *Tai Ping Sheng Hui Fang*; for instance, black bean soup for edema, apricot seed soup for cough. Adding spices to the maxim, Hu Si Hui, cook for the royal family during the Yuan Dynasty, wrote a book in which he recommended standards for meeting normal nutritional requirements. He added many recipes to his book, which was a first in diet and food therapy.[3]

The first book on pure botanical medicine (that is, not from animal or mineral sources) was produced in the fifteenth century. It was called *Jiu Huang Ben Cao* ("Medicine for Emergencies") and appeared in 1406. The author was Zhu Xiao (?–1425), whose keen interest in herbal medicine prompted him to commission people to survey various plants. From their reports, he selected those he wished to observe in his own garden. After dedicated research, he chose 414 edible specimens, including 276 that were new to the medical community, and recorded their names, preferred growth locations, shapes, sizes, properties, and taste, along with instructions for brewing. He then invited painters to make illustrations.

Zhen Nan Ben Cao appeared in 1476. Its author was Lan Mao (1397–1476), who was born in Yang Lin, Yunnan Province. A local pharmacopoeia, it contained some folk formulas among the more than four hundred herbal medicines it discussed. For some—Smilay glabra rhizoma and tendrilled fritillary bulb, for example—it was the first time these folk formulas had been recognized and included in medical research, as opposed to being handed down verbally from generation to generation.

Published in 1565, *Ben Cao Meng Quan*, written by Chen Jia Mo, was based on *Ben Cao Ji Yao* and the author's seven years of clinical experience. Some of the most popular herbal medicines used today are among the 742 recorded in this book, some for the first time. Another valuable contribution of this book is the discussion of storage techniques. It was recommended, for instance, to store herbs in a dry and cool environment, such as a sealed container that was buried.

Li Shi Zhen's *Ben Cao Gang Mu*

In Chinese medical history, *Ben Cao Gang Mu* by Li Shi Zhen (1518–1593) is an outstanding pharmacopoeia. It contains multiple contributions to Chinese culture and science and, through translation, has influenced medicine in many other parts of the world. A third-generation doctor, Li Shi Zhen began his studies as a child, reading his father's medical texts and following him as he practiced. When he was fourteen, at his father's urging, he took the national examination for government office. He passed the first stage but, after failing the subsequent stages, decided to dedicate himself to medicine. His reputation soared when, at age thirty, he cured the son of the royal family, who was suffering from a rare parasitic disease. He was invited by the Ming government to serve as a chief doctor in charge of medical and health events. Later, appointed president of the National Health Administration, his old dislike for the official life surfaced. He resigned after a year, citing poor health.

In his clinical practice, he discovered mistakes and shortcomings in the pharmacopoeias of his day, and resolved to write a new one. At age thirty-five, he began, and for the next twenty-seven years, he pored over thousands of medical books, going out to collect the herbs he did not plant himself. His research included observing and tasting some of the herbs first-hand. Relying on the foundations laid out in Tang Shen Wei's *Jing Shi Zheng Lei Ben Cao,* he finished his book in 1578, when he was sixty-two years old. He is also known to have written at least two other books, one concerning pulse diagnosis techniques and another concerning acupuncture and the theory of channels and collaterals.

Ben Cao Gang Mu's many contributions to medical science can be summarized as follows:

1. A summary of pharmacological knowledge before the sixteenth century. The book recorded 1,892 medicines, more than 10,000 formulas, and contained thousands of charts.

2. The most scientific classification system to date. The medicines were organized from "lower" to "super" class (from inorganic to organic, matching biological evolution). He also classified the medicines into sixty branches, under sixteen categories in total: water, fire, earth, metal and stone (mineral), grass, grain, vegetable, fruit, wood, cloth, warm, scale, shell, bird, beast (animal), and human. Every entry contained multiple subclassifications.

3. Correction of errors contained in previous pharmacopoeias.

4. Discussions pertaining to other sciences as well as medicine, including human physiology and pathology, clinical manifestations and symptoms of disease, botany, zoology, mineralogy, physics, astronomy, and meteorology.

Subsequent Pharmacopoeias

The publication of *Ben Cao Gang Mu* seemed to stimulate the publication of other medical texts, such as *Pao Zhi Da Fa*, published in 1622 and written by Liao Xi Yong (1556–1627?). This book specialized in pharmaceutical preparatory techniques. More than four hundred procedures were discussed. The preferred areas of growth, harvest times, ways to distinguish quality, materials used during preparation, the difference in properties after preparation, and contraindications were also included.

Ben Cao Bei Yao appeared in 1694. It was written by Wang Ang (1615–?), also called Ren An. Considering *Ben Cao Gang Mu* somewhat difficult to use in practice, he selected what he considered to be the most useful medicines and, in 460 entries, compiled a guidebook that became very popular in his day. Additions to this book appeared about sixty years later in the 1757 book *Ben Cao Cong Yin,* written by Wu Yi Luo. The author added 260 plants as well as ways in which to distinguish medicinal plants and prepare them for use.

Three physicians collaborated to write *De Pei Ben Cao,* which came out in 1761. They were Yan Xi Ting, Shi Zhan Ning, and Hong Ji An, and their book was based on the results of their original experiments. Based on *Ben Cao Gang Mu* insofar as classification was concerned, 647 medicines were listed. Special care was paid to interaction between medicines; for example, whether they counteracted each other, assisted each other increasing their effect, or whether a combination reduced effectiveness. The compatibility of medicines was the main concern of this book.

By the end of the eighteenth century, another expansion/revision of *Ben Cao Gang Mu* had appeared, authored by Zhao Xue Min (1719–1805). *Ben Cao Gang Mu Shi Yi* broadened the scope of medicinal resources by adding 716 medicines to those listed in the classic text. Zhao Xue Min spent forty years researching his book.

Zhi Wu Ming Shi Tu Kao, which appeared in 1848, can be found in the national library of many countries because of its important contributions to botany and medicine. The author was Wu Qi Jun (1789–1847), who traveled among many provinces in the course of his investigations. Devoted solely to botanic medicine, the book contains 1,700 entries (500 more than *Ben Cao Gang Mu*) as well as many valuable charts and illustrations.

Achievements in Formularization

Formularizations are unique to Chinese medicine, because medicines are almost always used in combination either to strengthen the effect or to control side effects. After long experience, Chinese pharmacologists have developed their own special and sophisticated methods for combining medicines.

As we have seen, formularization was initiated in the classic ancient text *Nei Jing* and followed up in other early texts. Those initial formulas, even though developed without any systematic theories, are still the primary formulas used in medicinal combinations in modern practice of Traditional Chinese Medicine. During the period between the Ming and Qing Dynasties (1368–1840 A.D.), formularization became an independent subject for symptomatic research. Theory became more complex, and a host of new combinations were invented. Among the many books published on the subject was *Pu Ji Fang*, written by Zhu Xiao, Professor Teng Shuo, and Liu Chun in the early days of the Ming. The most comprehensive book on formularization, it summarized the contents of most of the writings on formulas before the fifteen century and added new ones. When completed, it covered 2,175 categories and 61,000 formulas in depth. As an added bonus, much of the information included in this text came from ancient documents whose originals have been lost.

A very practical guide to formulas appeared in 1682. *Yi Fang Ji Jie*, written by Wang Ang, is a collection of 600 formulas divided into 21 categories, including diaphoretic, purgative, tonifying, energy regulators, wind dispersers, and draining damp. Formulas for emergency use were also included. Each category listing began with a brief description of and indications for that group of formulas, and each formula was accompanied by information on indications, composition, explanation, and commentary on modifications.

Progress in Research on Herbal Medicine in the Modern Era (1849–1949)

As exposure to Western medicine gradually increased in the nineteenth and twentieth centuries, Chinese physicians were faced with a challenge and an opportunity. The challenge was how to maintain the reputation and known efficacy of Chinese herbal medicines and medical techniques in the face of growing political opposition and the desire for modernization. The opportunity was to learn how to successfully combine the best features of Western and Chinese medicine for the benefit of the patient. Most of the population, especially in the rural areas and small cities, tended to rely on Chinese herbal medicine when they were sick. At this point in history, achievements in combining Western and Chinese medicine were still not significant, but a foundation was being built.

By 1920, small-scale research on the chemistry of herbal medicine and other pharmacological subjects was underway in China. In 1932, Chen Ke Hui discovered the pharmacological function of ephedrine—now a well-known medication for relieving the spasms of bronchial asthma.[4] More than forty different herbal medicines were investigated by Chen Ke Hui. This methodology greatly encouraged later scientists to use modern techniques to research other natural herbal medicines.

A physician named Zhang Xi Chun advocated combining Chinese and Western medical treatment modalities, believing them to be compatible. In his clinical practice, he observed how the two medical systems complemented each other and wrote about his experiences. He said, "Western medication is very good at controlling symptoms and is more focused on local problems. Chinese medication is more focused on finding the root cause of an illness and on treating the whole body. One is for result, one is for root cause. If we treat the difficult case by using western medication to treat Biao (clinical manifestation) and using Chinese medicine to treat the Ben (cause), the effect will be more significant."

Zhang Xi Chun created many interesting formulas in clinical practice, mixing Chinese herbal medicine together with Western drugs. He praised the temperature-reducing function of aspirin, for example, and felt it was a good medication for treating tuberculosis. He discovered, however, that its diaphoresis action is too strong for this condition and can hurt the Lung's Yin (fluid). A better treatment, he found, is to combine the use of aspirin with Xuan Shen (Scrophularia root) and Sha Shen (Glehnia root) "in order to tonify Lung's Yin, making it easier to cure the tuberculosis without any side-effects." This type of clinical research raised the pharmacology of Chinese herbal medicine to a higher level. For the first time, herbal medicine was being used not only to cure disease but to reduce side effects from the medicine itself.

Chinese doctors were beginning to wonder about why Chinese medicines work. Significant progress was made at this time in the areas of pharmacological function research, the grading of medicinal herbs, and formula theory, as scientists, dissatisfied with vague explanations and theories, used modern chemistry techniques to explore the essence and mystery of Chinese herbal medicine.

The Reediting of *Shen Nong Ben Cao Jing*

As previously mentioned, *Shen Nong Ben Cao Jing* was the earliest pharmacopoeia in Chinese medicine, but with the passing of time and political upheaval, the original text was lost. In 1844, a physician named Gu Guan Guang consulted references to this classic text in later books and republished *Shen Nong Ben Cao Jing*. This book was thought to be the best revision to date by contemporary doctors. In 1942, Liu Fu reedited *Shen Nong Ben Cao Jing* once more based upon Gu Guan Guang's book and others. Both books have special value for research in ancient medicine and pharmacopoeias.

A milestone in the attempt to reconcile Chinese medicine with Western medicine appeared in 1933 when, after many years researching *Shen Nong Ben Cao Jing* and Chinese pharmacology, Ruan Qi Yu selected 280 medicines from the 365 listed in *Shen Nong Ben Cao Jing*. Referring to his clinical experience, he explained the functions, indications, and properties of each medicine as they pertained to Western medical theory. He titled his book *Ben Cao Jing Xin Zhu*. Dosages, contraindications, and precautions for each medicine were also listed in detail. Ma Huang, for example, was explained as follows: "Due to the anti-bacterial function, it was recognized as having bitter properties; due to the diaphoresis ability it was thought of as warm medicine." And again: "This medicine can resolve the phlegm and soothe asthma, so it is very good for treating the acute bronchitis patient without sweat. But it is prohibited for the tuberculosis patient." At the same time, he emphasized that the functions of Chinese medicine could be verified only by long clinical use, and that using chemical analysis technique is not enough to determine a medicine's worth.

Research on Pharmacological Functions

Many pharmacological research texts appeared toward the end of the Qing Dynasty. In 1863, Tu Dao He wrote *Ben Cao Hui Cuan,* which was based on 20 previously published important pharmacopoeias. His book compiled 560 essential and popular medicines divided into 31 groups according to the function and property of the medicine: neutral tonic medicines, tonifying kidney medicine, dispersing cold medicine, clearing heat, cooling blood medicine, and so on. He included very precise information about the specific channel entered, indications, contraindications, and precautions for each medicine.

Representing a trend in utilizing the modern categorization technique was the pharmacological text *Zhui Xin Shi Yan Yao Wu Xue* (1933), written by Wen Jing Xiu. Working with a total of 400 medicines, the author categorized them into 23 groups: tonic medicines, digestion medicines, diuretic medicines, astringent medicines, and so on. Under each entry was listed the medicine's name, family, production source, effective/active component, property, function, indications, formulas (major combinations), contraindications, dosage, and other information.

The Grading of Herbal Medicines

As many false and inferior medicines began to flow into the pharmacological market, many doctors saw the necessity of identifying medicinal quality and dedicated themselves to this research. After many years of accumulating experience in this field, Zheng Xiao Yan summarized his findings on how to distinguish high-quality medicine from bad in his 1901 manuscript *Wei Yao Tiao Bian*. Later scholars carefully reedited the book, adding more information and their own experiences. In 1927, the book was published as *Zeng Ding Wei Yao Yiao Bian*. It became very popular and was considered the authoritative book on identifying medicinal quality. Here is one example:

> The best Ma Huang (Ephedra) is produced in Datong, Shanxi Province. It has a bulging look, with blue and yellow coloring on the outside and red coloring on the inside. The type grown in the northeast, having a thin and hard stem, is not used as medicine. Astraglus root is best when its color is white and slightly yellow; it has a sweet taste with a fresh soybean smell. If its skin color is dark red, its consistency hard, and has a taste like green grass, the quality is bad and odor should be very fragrant. Astralagus should be distinguished from wild ox horn and wild goat horn, for even though its color is black, inside there will be no pattern and there will be an offensive odor. These have no medicinal qualities.

This book played a very important role in controlling the quality of subsequent pharmacopoeias, because it instructed in proper identification procedures.

Formula Theory

Through centuries of clinical application and continual refinement, the theory of Chinese medicine grew more comprehensive. Formula theory was already an independent subject for research and had developed from pure experimentation. Researchers continued to refine basic principles and theories to explain existing formulas and to create new ones. Several collections of formulas created through experience were published, in which the theory of formulation was barely mentioned. The formula explanations also were often just transcribed anecdotally, from experience, without reference to the basic principles involved.

In the later part of the Qing Dynasty, researchers were beginning to realize that formulas should be used properly and flexibly; that is, once the basic meaning and principle of the formula is understood, it can be applied effectively. Aside from this trend, two major collections of formulas were published. One was *Gu Jin Yi Fang Ji Cheng* (1936) compiled by Wu Ke Qian. Based on 170 older formula books, he systematically arranged and categorized over ten thousand formulas in this book. Also included were the contents of 160 ancient formula books, which have since been lost. This book was considered the encyclopedia of medicinal formulas at that time. The other major collection was a comprehensive medical book that included 470 formulas as treatments for conditions in gynecology, internal medicine, pediatrics, and ophthalmology. In the general introduction, the basic theory of formulation is discussed, and it is emphasized that interrelation and compatibility among the medicines in a formula are the key to its effectiveness.

In the modern period, two significant texts combined medical formulas from the Chinese and Western systems. They were Ding Fu Bao's *Zhong Xi Yi Fang Hui Tong* (1910) and Chen Ji Wu's *Zhong Xi Yan Fang Xin Bian* (1916). Dr. Chen and Dr. Ding both traveled to Japan to study Western medicine. They claimed that both traditions have their virtues and faults, even in medicinal formulation, and that it is necessary to combine the two formula techniques.

An example of the combined treatment of Western and Chinese medicine is the method used to address bronchopneumonia in children. Since the disease is caused by a bacterial and viral infection during a period of low physical resistance, the doctors use herbal medicines, traditional methods of massage along the spinal column (Nie Ji therapy) to increase the digestive function, and acupuncture and injections into needling points to increase the patient's appetite, raising nutrition levels and therefore body resistance. Antibiotics are used to combat inflammation of the lung in severe cases. Clinical trials have verified that this combination therapy has brought major improvements over and above the simple administration of antibiotics.

Although contemporary doctors practicing Traditional Chinese Medicine are trained to have a thorough working knowledge of how to use herbal medicines most effectively, pharmacology as a specialty has been growing in the last forty years. These professional pharmacists assure quality control, and their continuing study of the art of herbal medicine is constantly adding to the knowledge of their forebears.

Notes

1. The "messenger" medicine is the substance whose sole purpose is to guide the activating medicine to its intended target; for instance, if a doctor prescribes a medicine for treating a disease of the liver, he will add a messenger medicine to guide the curing medicine to the liver.
2. Many ancient writers used "auspicious numbers," such as five or three; in most cases, the use of one of these numbers in theoretical writing means simply "many."
3. Predating his work was a Mongolian folk therapy recorded in *The Secret History of Mongolia*: horse milk wine. This treatment was recognized prior to the Yuan Dynasty as effective for reviving a patient from a faint caused by heavy bleeding.
4. Now ephedrine is manufactured synthetically, but its original form was an extract from the Chinese medicine Ma Huang and the herb ephedra.

6

Sea, River, Stream, Spring, Well: The History of Acupuncture and Moxibustion

Acupuncture and moxibustion are the application of fine needles or heat, respectively, to various points on the body—called acupoints—in order to cure disease. The various acupoints are located by the doctor based on his knowledge of the theory of channels and meridians (discussed in chapter 1). The fine points of these techniques were developed over many centuries in China, first simply passed down from doctors to their apprentices, and later systematized in medical schools.

Acupuncture, the channel and meridian theory, and some needling manipulation techniques are first mentioned in the classic medical book of Traditional Chinese Medicine, the *Nei Jing*. The material in this classic medical text actually dates much earlier—some say, all the way back to the second of the "celestial emperors," Huang Di, who may have lived as early as the 25th century B.C. and is credited with many medical discoveries, including acupuncture. It is certainly the case that the acupuncture techniques discussed in the *Nei Jing* were in use long before the actual publication date of the book, as attested to by references in the book to many earlier works, now lost.

Acupuncture theory was rooted on the basic Chinese medical theory. There are organs and meridians (channels), which connect the organs and tissue together and help the distribution and transportation of nutrients to every part of the body. This basic fundamental theory was well established in *Nei Jing*. *Nei Jing* is the oldest and most comprehensive medical book. It was divided into two parts/volumes. One was named *Su Wen* (Plain question); another was named *Ling Shu* (Spiritual Axial). The first paragraph of *Ling Shu* is about nine needles and twelve sources. The nine needles include:

Chan Needle—1.6 inches in length
Yuan Needle—1.6 inches in length
Ti Needle—3.5 inches in length
Feng Needle—1.6 inches in length
Pi Needle—4 inches in length, 0.2 inch in width
Yuan Li Needle—1.6 inches in length
Hao Needle—3.6 inches in length
Chang Needle—7 inches in length
Da Needle—4 inches in length

Each needle has its own shape and is used for a different purpose. Before these needles were invented, the sharp stones, bamboo needle, wood needle, bone needle and bronze needle had been used for a long long time. But now many of the above mentioned nine needles were not used in clinical practice. Some of the needles have been replaced by new surgical tools. What we use often in practice are Hao needles and Chang needles. Hao means small; Chang means long. The stainless steel needles we use in daily acupuncture. Mei Hua Needle, also called plum blossom needle, looks like a small hammer. On the hammer head there are seven small, short needles which are most often used for skin problems such as eczema. The auricular needle is used on the ear. It is also called the subcutaneous needle.

In explaining how acupuncture can cure the disease, it was said, acupuncture can open the meridian; it can regulate the blood and energy flow; it can balance the Yin and Yang.

Acupuncture theory has not improved much since the *Nei Jing*. The needle itself, however, has developed very much with the advance of the industry.

There are two difficult aspects in performing acupuncture. One is how to choose the point to insert the needle; the second is how to manipulate the needle to make sure you send the right needle in the points. About these two parts, *Nei Jing* also has a brilliant description. It really puzzled the historians, how the ancient doctor knew so much. Some even wondered if this science might have come from a person from outside the planet. But the truth is, all the knowledge came from the ancient doctor's huge clinical practice and clinical trials.

Since the *Nei Jing*, there were many special books and medical documents about acupuncture and moxibustion published.

The first book devoted entirely to acupuncture was written during the Jin Dynasty (265–420 A.D.) by a man who started his career as a historian. Huang Fu Mi (215–282 A.D.), born in Gansu province, became a great author and historian with numerous publications to his credit. In his mid-forties, Huang contracted severe arthritis and suffered subsequent paralysis. He underwent a course of acupuncture treatment and was not only cured by felt rejuvenated. From that time on, he devoted himself to medical research. Although the Jin rulers invited him several times to serve in the government (a post that would have given him great status and a certain amount of security), he refused in order to continue his own research projects. Summarizing the accumulated knowledge of acupuncture and adding his own clinical experience, he wrote a book that became a standard text in medical schools centuries later. *Zhen Jiu Jia Yi Jing* ("The ABCs of Acupuncture and Moxibustion") was published sometime between 256 and 282 A.D.

Zhen Jiu Jia Yi Jing is a treatise outlining the number of acupoints, their location, and needle manipulation procedure.

It also lists, for each acupoint, a practical list of indications of use. Due to the author's excellent literary style, this book turned out to be a concise, well-written, practical basis for learning acupuncture then and in the future, in China and in other countries, such as Japan and Korea. This book is still studied today by students of Traditional Chinese Medicine.

The next major push in the field of acupuncture appeared during the Tang Dynasty (618–906). Most of the important books on the subject were summarized in Sun Si Miao's *Qian Jin Yao Fang*. Sun[1] was the first doctor to discover the function of the Ashi point, a tender place that may appear not in the normal meridian point but anywhere on the body. This point can be needled to treat whatever problem arises.

The Tang rulers were the first to establish a government-run National Health Administration, which set standards and trained doctors in a systematic, three-year program. The National Health Administration had a special department for the study of acupuncture, which was staffed by doctors, assistants, and technicians who specialized in acupuncture technique. Every medical student was required to read Huang Fu Mi's basic text *Zhen Jiu Jia Yi Jing*.

The casting of two bronze statues as a teaching tool for acupuncture students was one of the greatest achievements in the healing arts during the Song Dynasty (960–1279). In the year 1027, a life-sized model of the adult male form was produced, from which were cast two bronze statues, which could be disassembled. Replicas of the internal organs were installed inside. The meridians (channels) and 657 acupoints were carved into each surface. When used for teaching and testing, the surface of a model was waxed and water stored inside the acupoints. If a needle was inserted at the correct point, the water would leak out.

The statues were accompanied by a text, *Xin Zhu Zhen Jiu Tong Ren Tu Jing*, ("Classic Chart on the New Bronze Acupuncture Statues") written by Wang Wei Yi, which describes 657 acupoints. (As many of these points appear on both sides of the body, there are actually only 354 different acupoints in total.) The first and second volumes of this book describe the location of the acupoints as well as the routes of the twelve channels and the two "extra-meridian" channels, Du and Ren (Du runs along the spine, Ren along the midline of the front of the body). The third volume discusses the function of the acupoints according to their position in the body. As a testament to its worth, passages from this book were carved in stone and placed as a monument on the campus of one of the government-sponsored universities of the time.[2]

Additional discoveries about the technique and its applications were documented by other authors during the progressive Song Dynasty. The first book to advocate the selection of acupoints according to syndrome was *Zhen Jiu Zi Sheng Jing* ("Classic on Rejuvenation with Acupuncture and Moxibustion"). Written in 1165 by a doctor named Wang Zhi Zhong, the book first described and indicated forty-six charts the acupoints in the head, chest, abdomen, and limbs according to the route of their meridians. Several of these points were new discoveries by this author. In addition to acupuncture, Wang's book discussed the manipulation of the acupuncture needles and—for the first time—the technique of moxibustion (the application of heat at the acupuncture points). Moxibustion proved to be an especially effective technique for the treatment of tuberculosis, hemorrhoids, diarrhea, dysentery, athlete's foot, carbuncles, night blindness, and palsy, as well as in the slowing of the aging process.[3] Moxibustion techniques, point location, and contraindications for moxibustion were also discussed. The final section of Wang's text prescribed the correct acupoints for 193 diseases and syndromes, including those afflicting the reproductive, urinary, and digestive systems.

The author's discovery of two more points for the urinary bladder channel and one more point for the gall bladder channel, as well as eighteen others, were of significant value and added to the basics previously laid down in *Xin Zhu Tong Ren Zhen Jiu Tu Jing*.

Locating the Correct Acupoints
One outstanding contribution made by Wang Zhi Zhong was his use of the "Tong Shen Cun" as the standard "inch" for calibrating acupoint location. Used to this day, this unit is equal to the lengths of the second joint of the patient's index finger, which, of course, differs from person to person. This and additional guidelines for the accurate location of the acupoints, necessary for achieving good therapeutic results, were meticulously recorded by Wang, who stressed the importance of finding the "tender point" (sensitive point on the body) and also recognized that the patient's body position is important in locating the acupoint. If the body position is varied, the point location will be different.

Another milestone in the history of acupuncture was *Biao You Fu* ("Poem to Illustrate the Deepest Secrets"), written by Dou Mo (1190–1280). Dou Mo became a high official in the government as well as an expert in both literature and acupuncture. He was known for his method of point selection based on channel differentiation, as opposed to differentiation according to Zang Fu (internal organs), the prevailing method of the time. In channel differentiation, the doctor observes the patient's complaints and clinical manifestation—including complexion, pulse, and so on—to determine which channel is involved; the acupoints concerned with that particular channel are then manipulated to cure the problem.

It was Dou Mo's practice to employ the five shu points below the elbows and knees—jing (well), ying (spring), shu (stream), jing (river), and he (sea)[4]—as a way of understanding how energy flows in the body, which would guide the choice of acupoints in clinical practice. *Biao You Fu* was well researched, as its references to earlier texts show. It was written in poetic form as a mnemonic device, so as to be more easily learned and used by medical students. This book was the clearest explanation yet of the way in which acupuncture can affect the flow of blood and Qi (energy) along the meridians of the body.

Two great contributions to the practice of acupuncture were made less than a hundred years later by a doctor named Hua Shou. His book, *Shi Si Jing Fa Hui* ("The Enhancement of 14 Channels") was published in 1341. Doctor Hua researched the theory of channels and collaterals and pointed out the difference between Ren, Du, and six other extra channels. (The Du and Ren meridians have their own points along the front and back of the body; added to the twelve regular channels, that adds up to fourteen channels altogether.)

Secondly, based on the two ancient texts *Su Wen* and *Ling Shu*, Doctor Hua verified the 657 acupoints, differentiated the Yin from the Yang acupoints, and he defined the location of acupoints using bones as landmarks.

About this time in history, a theory arose that originally caused a great deal of controversy but which eventually was recognized as valid and contributed to the increasing sophistication of acupuncture treatment. This theory argued that the time of day should be one of the factors considered in selection of acupoints. According to this theory, some acupoints open or close at certain times. If a needle is inserted on a closed point, the treatment will be useless. This theory is not practical in all cases, but some doctors agree with its effectiveness.

Milestones in the Development of Moxibustion

The first record of a female physician is a doctor known as Chun Yu Yan, who lived during the Han Dynasty (202 B.C.–220 A.D.). It is recorded that she was called to the palace to treat the queen, to whom she administered a pill composed of aconite.

Bao Gu, wife of Dr. Ge Hong, was a well-known specialist in moxibustion therapy during the Jin Dynasty (265–420 A.D.). We know of her through a biography recorded in a history of the Jin Dynasty—though all information about her is indirect. Bao Gu invented a treatment for warts using moxa that was remarkably effective. She trained many students in the moxibustion treatment as well. So great was the people's respect for this doctor and teacher that they raised a memorial statue of her on Guang Zhou Yue Xiu Mountain, which is still in place today.

Another advocate of moxibustion was Wang Tao, who introduced many different moxibustion techniques in his book *Wai Tai Mi Yao* ("Essential Secrets from the Master's Podium") during the Tang Dynasty.

Emergency care via moxibustion was the topic undertaken by Wei Ren Shi Nian in his book *Bei Ji Jiu Fa* ("Emergency Moxibustion Techniques"), which was published in 1226. Charts illustrated how to use moxibustion to treat heart congestion, toothache, acute laryngitis, cholera, abscess of the intestines, carbuncle, and cellulitis, among others. Because of the many new techniques for emergency care first mentioned in this book, *Bei Ji Jiu Fa* holds an important position in the history of the moxibustion technique.

The beginning of the Yuan Dynasty (1260–1368) marked the unification of China by the Mongols. Communication between China and Mongolia had been going on for some time, including exchange of medical theories and techniques. The Mongolians contributed a unique moxibustion technique: a heating pad made of wool carpet soaked in butterfat mixed with fennel. (Fennel is a very "hot-property" medicine that improves blood circulation in order to expel the cold from the body.) Bloodletting to expel pathogens was another well-known traditional Mongolian therapy that was not practiced by Chinese doctors, although it was widely used in the West during the Middle Ages.

During the Ming Dynasty (1368–1644), acupuncture and moxibustion progressed under the benevolent encouragement of the government. In 1443, the Ming government ordered the casting of acupuncture models, imitating the Song style (see p. 78). An increasing number of specialty books on acupuncture and moxibustion were published, many of which included detailed charts.

One of the most significant was *Zhen Jiu Ju Ying* ("Superior Acupuncture and Moxibustion Techniques") published in 1529 by Gao Wu, who lived in Zhejiang Province. He was a versatile doctor, especially skilled in acupuncture and moxibustion. Gao collected the theories and clinical examples from sixteen different texts on acupuncture and moxibustion and added the results of his own experiences. He criticized some views that he believed were superstitious, such as the belief that one could not insert needles in certain points, or evil would be released. Recognizing the difference of point location in male, female, and child, he designed and had cast three bronze statues as a standard for point location.

The current text on acupuncture and moxibustion for medical students is based on a book written by Yang Ji Zhou in 1601, called *Zhen Jiu Da Cheng* ("Significant Achievements in Acupuncture and Moxibustion"). Referring to his family's secret records and his own clinical experience, Yang described channel theory, point location, and the manipulation techniques for needle and moxibustion along with their indications. He stressed the necessity for, and described his successful experience with, combining acupuncture and herbal medicine. Some clinical case studies were meticulously recorded. This book is a model for research, because the author recorded not only the successful cases, but also the unsuccessful ones, and included his analysis as to why a treatment did or did not work. Some older acupuncture documents were kept in circulation because of this book's reference to them.

During the middle of the Qing Dynasty (1644–1912), acupuncture and moxibustion suffered a setback when the feudal government decided that needles and moxibustion with fire were not suitable treatment for the emperor, and issued an order in 1822 banning the department of acupuncture and moxibustion in the Royal Health Administration forever. This ban was strictly enforced in the central health agency, but because the techniques were so effective and well-known throughout China, they were never completely prohibited for the rest of the population.

In fact, during the next hundred years, over a hundred books on the techniques of acupuncture and moxibustion, the theory of meridians and collaterals, the prescriptions of acupoints for many common diseases, contraindications of acupuncture, the correct way to use the index finger joint as a unit of measurement to find the acupoint, energy flow theory, and many other topics made their way into print, and research continued.

Zhong Guo Zhen Jiu Zhi Liao Xue ("Chinese Acupuncture and Moxibustion Therapy"), published in 1931, was the first book to use as a reference the discoveries in anatomy and physiology by Western medicine. It was written by Cheng Dan An, who collected the theories of many well-known doctors and combined them with his own clinical experience. His book also discussed the use of acupuncture and moxibustion in the treatment of disease in many specialty areas, such as gynecology, pediatrics, and internal medicine, and included some case studies. Cheng's book became a valuable reference book for acupuncture research.

Another significant text that appeared in 1933 was *Zhen Jiu Cuan Yao* ("Essential Collection of Acupuncture and Moxibustion Techniques"). What made this work special were its color charts of the meridians and acupoints, its descriptions of the local anatomy of acupoints, and its many beautiful and easily remembered poems for learning a point location, indications, and meridian routes. This is a very good book for beginning acupuncture students, and it is still in use today.

Acupuncture and moxibustion were at first discouraged by the government in the early twentieth century under a regime that increasingly advocated study of Western medical science. However, under the leadership of Mao Ze Dong, a firm believer in the traditional therapies, Chinese medicine was restored to its former status. Today, acupuncture is a respected treatment that is often used in conjunction with Western techniques in China. The first Western studies of acupuncture involved its use as a replacement for chemical anaesthesia during surgery (first brought to the attention of the American public by journalist James Reston in the mid-1960s at the beginning of China's "open-door" policy). Western physicians are increasingly respectful of this aspect of Chinese medicine, although it has yet to become a standard recommendation for treatment. A hopeful sign is that a few insurance companies now reimburse patients for acupuncture treatment.

Notes

1. More about Sun Si Miao's many contributions to Chinese Medicine may be found in chapter 5.
2. This monument is still in place in Beijing at a national university campus.
3. Moxibustion is believed to slow the aging process by improving blood circulation.
4. These points are given names corresponding to bodies of water because the meridians appeared to early doctors like irrigation channels, or like a system of waterways where the smaller streams merge into larger ones.

7

Preventive Medicine: The Cornerstone of Traditional Chinese Medicine

One thing that has never changed in the practice of Chinese medicine throughout the ages is its examination of the entire person in diagnosing and treating disease and in recommending a healthy lifestyle. As early as the *Nei Jing*, the effect of mental and emotional states on pathology, pathogenesis, and recovery was recognized. It was believed that positive attitudes and a pleasant social environment could reduce the disease rate. Ahead of its time, the ancient *Nei Jing* also advocated the prevention of disease through physical exercise.

A proper diet was also recommended throughout history as a way to prevent illness and, sometimes, to heal it. There are records of ancient courts employing a dietitian whose sole job was to choose proper medical food for the emperor. Diet was prescribed, not only according to its healing properties, but was also chosen according to season and other qualities.

Chinese proverb:
The superior doctor prevents illness; the mediocre doctor cures imminent illness; the inferior doctor treats actual illness.

The great doctor Hua Tuo (148–208 A.D.) invented a routine of special exercise for prevention of disease. One exercise, named Wu Qin Xi (five animals exercise—based on the movements of the tiger, deer, bear, monkey, and bird), promoted movement in the head, torso, waist, and all four limbs. It is reported that two of Hua Tuo's students, Wu Pu and Fan E, were great proponents of this exercise. They practiced this exercise continuously and lived remarkably long and healthy lives. The five animals exercise is an essential part of the exercise, breathing, and meditation program known as Qi Gong, which reached its zenith in popularity during the Ming-Qing period (1368–1912).

Qi Gong was originally developed as an aid to longevity. It was influenced by the Daoist belief that special breathing exercises could prolong life, and by the meditation techniques of Buddhism, which advocated quieting the mind—also believed to contribute to longevity. In 1442 Leng Qian wrote a book called *Xiu Ling Yao Zhi* ("The Key to Longevity") to introduce people to methods for regulating and taking care of the body to adapt to the changes of the four seasons. It included several new special physical and breathing exercise techniques, such as the sixteen Duan Jin (precious steps), the eight Duan Jin, and Dao Yin Que Bing Fa (Dao Yin means "gentle movement" and Que Bing means "prevent disease"). *Xiu Ling Yao Zhi* was written in a poetic style so as to be easily remembered. Here is an example, a poem for longevity:

When inhaling Qi is elevated to umbilicus,
at the same time make a swallowing movement,
which helps the water meet fire.
Turning the tongue to produce saliva fluid,
swallowing it down to Dan Tian, frequently and smoothly,
practice this day after day
for longevity and health.

This poem emphasizes the importance of Yin-Yang balance in the preservation of health.

The History of Vaccination

Infectious diseases puzzled physicians for centuries. History records outbreaks of chicken pox, for instance, in many areas worldwide; it was first recorded in China around the 4th century B.C. Because of the damage chicken pox caused and its contagious nature, doctors searched for a way to control it. The Tang Dynasty text *Qian Jin Yao Fang* ("A Thousand Golden Necessary Formulas") by the famous doctor Sun Si Miao recorded some medicinal formulas designed to prevent and treat chicken pox, but it was not until the invention of the vaccination that an effective preventive method was discovered.

In 1884, two authors investigating the history of vaccinations examined old records and reported that the first medical record of vaccination appeared in the early part of the Tang Dynasty, citing a doctor named Zhao, who had first used the technique. The next historical mention of the technique tells of an unnamed doctor who successfully vaccinated the son of the premier against chicken pox during the later Song Dynasty (960–1279).

The complete vaccination technique was recorded in detail in two books published in 1695 and 1742. There were two different techniques. One was named Dou Yi Fa, which means "let people wear the patient's clothes." Because the patient's clothes are contaminated with the seepage of the rash (chicken pox), it can induce the production of immunity to the disease. This method was primary and not very effective or safe. The second technique, named Bi Miao Fa (nasal vaccination), was performed three different ways. First was Jiang Miao Fa, which placed a cotton ball dipped in the seepage of the chicken pox rash into the nose of an uninfected person. Second was Han Miao Fa (dryness), which collected the scars of a chicken pox patient, ground them into a powder, and then administered the powder to an uninfected person through the nose. The third was Shui Miao Fa (water), where the powder was prepared as before, but mixed with water and soaked in a cotton ball, which was placed in the nose of an uninfected person. The second and third techniques were the most effective.

Zhong Dou Xin Shu recorded significant results. In vaccinating nine thousand people, only twenty or thirty developed an infection. The Qing Emperor Kang Xi recorded in his chronicles in 1666, "The Government ordered the people to receive the vaccination, and all vaccinated people got a good result." Known as a great emperor in Chinese history, in this case he did take care of his people's health.

This now-famous preventive treatment for infectious disease lay dormant for the next hundred years until the British physician Edward Jenner rediscovered the technique in 1796, using the cowpox virus to vaccinate effectively against smallpox.

III
Clinical Medicine

8
Internal Medicine

The most ancient book on medicinal plants, *Shan Hai Jing* ("Hill and Sea Classic"), which could have been written as early as 700 B.C., describes a number of different diseases, such as lump, hemorrhoid, carbuncle, cellulitis, paralysis, malaria, mania, and epidemic disease. It was already being recognized by Chinese doctors that some external symptoms can indicate diseases that occur inside the body.

The doctor Hua Tuo (148–208 A.D.), an early specialist in internal medicine as well as in surgery, acupuncture, gynecology, and pediatrics, exercised the principle that one disease can be treated with several different methods and that differing diseases can be treated with the same medicine. For example, in the book *San Guo Zhi* ("History of Three Kingdoms"), Hua Tuo recorded two cases with identical symptoms: headache and fever. After examination, Hua Tuo diagnosed that one patient suffered interior excess, but the other suffered exterior excess. He then used purgative therapy for the first patient and diaphoresis therapy for the second. Both achieved cures.

Hua's contemporary Zhang Zhong Jin wrote a landmark text on internal medicine, *Shang Han Za Bing Lun* ("Treatise on Febrile Disease Caused by Cold and the Miscellaneous Diseases"). His principles for classification of symptoms are still in use today in clinical practice. (For more on Zhang's theories, see chapter 1).

A total of 784 internal diseases were recorded in the twenty-seven volumes of *Zhu Bing Yuan Hou Lun* ("Treatise on the Source and Manifestation of Many Diseases"), written in 610 by Cao Yuan Fang. This book stands out by its very detailed etiology and clinical records. Cao outlined preventative and therapeutic measures to be taken for many infectious diseases, such as thread worm, pediculosis, and leprosy.

On the pathology of athlete's foot, Cao Yuan Fang pointed out that this complaint was related to the eating of white rice over a long period of time. He predicted that eating the chaff of rice could prevent athlete's foot and prescribed treatment consisting of eating pig liver, red and black beans, and Job's tears seed. It is now known that all four are rich in Vitamin B, which is a very effective cure for this problem.

More research on the problem of athlete's foot was contributed in 1093 by Dong Ji, who described the pathogen, clinical manifestations, and treatment for the disease. He claimed that there were imbalances of Yin and Yang (deficiency and excess) in patients suffering from this disease. Offering forty-six formulas for treatment, he advised different treatments at different seasons. Dryness and humidity of the patient's environment, he said, as well as the strength and age of the patient, should be considered.

Mental diseases had been described as early as the *Nei Jing*. Now appeared the book *Qian Jin Yao Fang* ("Ten Thousand Essential Golden Formulas"), written by Sun Si Miao[1] in approximately 640, which addressed psychiatric diseases in much greater detail. The clinical manifestations of mania, depression, anxiety, and many other states were noted. Epilepsy was described in terms of the blue color of the nose and mouth, convulsions, lolling of the tongue, and shaking of the head.

Several texts dating from this period show that knowledge of diabetes was proceeding rapidly. It was noted by one doctor, for example, that the urine of diabetes patients was sweet. *Qian*

Jin Yao Fang suggested diet therapy for many diseases, such as diabetes, edema, and liver disease. A third text proposed the use of white fabric to test a diabetic patient's urine. If no staining was detected, then the problem was thought to be cured.

During the Song and Yuan Dynasties (960–1368), significant progress was made in internal medicine, both in theory and in clinical practice. The National Health Administration of the Song included a department of Feng (Wind Syndrome) diseases, which included strokes and diseases marked by tremors. A very comprehensive medical text differentiating the various Wind Syndrome diseases was authorized and published by the Song government in 1111–1117. Another significant text published during this period recognized edema as being of several types and accompanied each with a series of therapies.

Tuberculosis was the topic of Ge Ke Jiu, who wrote *Shi Yao Shen Shu* in 1348. He created ten very effective formulas designed to treat bleeding and coughing, and to rebuild the body by tonifying (increasing energy). This book is still a standard text for Traditional Chinese Medicine physicians studying and treating tuberculosis.

Dermatology

During this period (Ming-Qing), the first book on leprosy appeared. Entitled *Jie Wei Yuan Shu* ("Techniques for Treating Leprosy"), it was written by a doctor named Shen Zhi Wen in 1550. In his book, Shen distilled the essence of the research and investigation done by his father and grandfather, who were both physicians, and added his own clinical experience. His comprehensive book discussed pathogenisis, epidemics, clinical manifestation, contagious characteristics, therapy, and prevention of the disease. He introduced his method of treating leprosy with

Da Feng Zi (seed of Hydnocarpus anthelmintica pier), and he corrected some current erroneous ideas about the therapy.

Syphilis and its causes were recognized during this period as well. The first medical text specifically devoted to the subject was written by a doctor named Chen Si Cheng, who also benefited from studying the research of former generations as well as years of his own experience. Chen Si Cheng concluded, correctly, that syphilis is not only spread from direct contact (such as sexual intercourse) but also by congenital and indirect means. In his writings, he recorded the clinical manifestations of the disease and recommended treatment with the herbal medicines Dan Sha (Mercury) and Xiong Huang (As_2S_2).

During the Ming and Qing Dynasties (1368–1912), the development of internal medicine was characterized by the appearance of many new sophisticated and practical medical hypotheses brought about by vigorous debate and discussion. A great deal of clinical and diagnostic research on internal diseases and syndromes was summarized and published. Two primary theories were being disputed among the different schools: 1) Wen Bu (warm and tonifying) theory, and 2) Xiang Huo (Premier Heat) theory.

The Wen Bu (Warm and Tonifying) Theory

The symbolic apologists of the Wen Bu school were Xue Ji, Zhang Jie Bin, and Zhao Xian Ke. All of them disapproved of the overuse of cold and cool medicines to counteract Kidney Yang. They believed that life is centered in the Kidney Yang and that every organ needs Kidney Yang to perform its proper function. They therefore emphasized the importance of Kidney Yang in the preservation of health and reflected this viewpoint in their writing.

Xue Ji (1488–1558) lived in Jiangsu Province. He was well educated with a strong background in Chinese medicine. His father had served as president of the Royal Health Administration. Xue published many books on the subject of internal medicine, and his primary concerns were the deficiency of Zhen Yin (original Yin) and Zhen Yang (original Yang). Xue Ji also had considerable clinical experience in treating gynecological, pediatric, and ophthalmic diseases. One of his many publications was a compilation of his medical case histories.

Zhang Jie Bin (1563–1640) succeeded Xue Ji as a proponent of the Wen Bu school. He was born and lived in Zhejiang Province, but he followed his father to Beijing and studied the art of medicine while still a child. He served in the army for a short while as a secretary, thereafter devoting his life to the research and practice of Chinese medicine.

Zhang Jie Bin theorized that Zhen Yang deficiency was rare or nonexistent, but that deficiency of Zhen Yin was common. He believed that it was very important to warm and tonify Kidney Yang and Kidney Yin, and to avoid damage to the kidney from cool and cold herbal medicine. He created many useful and effective medicinal formulas for tonifying the kidney, although, based on his reputation, later doctors often tended to overuse these medicines, believing incorrectly that "if some is good, more is better." Late in life, Zhang compiled his clinical experiences into a book, which was published in 1640. This work was a comprehensive encyclopedia containing medical theory, diagnosis, therapeutic principles, comments, clinical experiences, *materia medica*, and his own experiences and explanations.

Zhang's observations of some disease processes, such as the manifestation of stroke, showed great insight. Chinese medicine traditionally related stroke to wind, and named it Zhong Feng, which means "attacked by wind." Zhang was of the opinion that the syndrome was not related to exogenous wind and cold, but resulted from interior damage.

The third important proponent of the Wei Bu theory was Zhao Xian Ke, who lived in 1687. His contribution was the Ming Men (Life Gate) theory, wherein he stated that the Life Gate is the source of life and emphasized the importance of "Life Gate fire." This theory was essential to all of his beliefs about the preservation of health and clinical practice, and based on his theory, many excellent formulas were developed to tonify Kidney Yang for the treatment of Deficiency Chronic Diseases.

In science, it is important not to overemphasize any one theory, because no one theory explains everything. The Wen Bu theory came under criticism by several doctors during the late Qing Dynasty (seventeenth and eighteenth centuries) who believed that it was unwise to overuse pungent and hot medicine to tonify, irrespective of the differentiation of syndrome.

Professional Diseases Analyzed During the Ming

During the Ming Dynasty, as industry prospered under a relatively stable government, mineral exploration, cast iron, textile and dyeing businesses caused many different professional diseases, and gradually more and more knowledge of professional disease and experience were accumulated.

Xue Ji recorded one typical professional disease, that of a silversmith, in his book of case studies. The silversmith was always handling silver and other raw minerals, and suffered from fatigue, alternating hot and cold flashes, and numbness. In the beginning, doctors mistook this as a carbuncle, and prescribed oral administration of cold medicine, without result. Xue Ji thought this case was caused by a toxic reaction to overexposure to silver. He suggested that the proper procedure would be to increase the patient's resistance and flush the toxin from his body. He prescribed tonifying herbs to be taken orally and frequent hand washing. His diagnosis and treatment were proven out when the patient was indeed cured.

There were very detailed records in *Ben Cao Gang Mu* (1578 A.D.) about lead poisoning in mine workers. Close proximity to the toxin and stagnant air contributed to sallow, yellow skin, abdominal distention and poor appetite, and, in the worst case, death.

Many reports of carbon monoxide poisoning were recorded in the Ming Dynasty. *Ben Cao Gang Mu* and *Jing Yue Quan Shu* both mentioned that carbon monoxide can cause coma and death. Many preventive measures were suggested, such as using bamboo tubes to induce the carbon monoxide out of coal mines and houses. Other suggestions were that people who work in mines must switch their job after two years, noting that the workers will lose hair and eyebrows due to the toxic buildup of mercury.

Xiang Huo Theory (Premier Heat)

Many comprehensive medical texts appeared during the Ming and Qing Dynasties, among them *Yi Xue Zheng Zhuan* ("Biography in Medical Format") written in about 1500 A.D. by Yu Tuan (1438–1517), who lived in Zhejiang Province. This text covered internal medicine, gynecology, traumatology, and pediatrics. The author was a follower of the theory of Zhu Dan Xi and included his theory first under the entry for each disease, followed by the opinions of other doctors. More than a thousand medicinal formulas were recorded in this book.

Ming Yi Za Zhu ("Miscellaneous Commentaries by a Well-Known Doctor"), written in 1549 by Wang Lun, had the distinction of applying several theories to different diseases. In his summary of internal medical theory, Wang advocated following the theories of Zhang Zhong Jing when treating exterior syndrome; the teachings of Li Gao for interior injury diseases; the theories of Liu Wan Su when treating the feverish diseases; and the principles of Zhu Dan Xi for the treatment of miscellaneous diseases. Wang Lun was of the opinion that absorbing the virtues of different theories and doctors increased the effectiveness of treatments. This work contributed greatly to a restoration of balance to Chinese medical treatments.

An interesting discussion of the prevention of stroke appears in a book written in 1615 by Gong Ting Xian, who served with his father in the Royal Health Administration. He stated: "Before the stroke attacks, there are always some preceding symptoms. If the patient feels numbness in the thumb or a tingling sensation, or lack of strength in the hands or feet, or muscular tremors, stroke will occur during the following three years. The patient should take Liu Wei Di Huang Wan in the morning and Zhi Li Zhi Shu Wan and Sou Feng Shun Qi Wan in the evening. By taking these medicines consistently, over time this disease can be cured." His book also contained sections of medicine specific to geriatric problems.

Zheng Yin Mai Zhi ("Symptom, Pathogen, Pulse, and Therapy") published in 1641, was written by Qin Jing Ming and Qin Huang Shi. Based on the work of Zhu Dan Xi, it took thirty years to compile. The authors changed the way in which the information on internal diseases was organized from Zhu Dan Xi's classification by pulse, which they felt was confusing, to a system that the authors believed would be more practical in the clinical setting.

Besides these general texts, many specialty texts were published during the Ming and Qing period, including texts on tuberculosis, deficiency disease, malaria, stroke, and even the clinical manifestations of liver cirrhosis and abdominal cancer.

Yi Lin Gai Cuo ("Correction of Some Mistakes in the Medical Field") was written in 1830 by Wang Qing Ren. The main contribution of this book is the establishment of the therapeutic principles of Tonifying Blood, Moving Blood, and Dispersing

Blood Stasis in treating the diseases of internal medicine. Many of the formulas he created for moving blood and dispersing blood stasis are still in use today.

Fei Bo Xiong was a well-regarded doctor in 1865. "There are many different diseases in clinical practice," he stated, "but they can be classified into two types: exterior and interior syndromes. For the deficiency syndrome, tonifying can balance it; for excess syndrome, reducing can calm the overactivity to return the body to homeostasis. The harmonizing principle is very simple, but it is also miraculous." Based on this thinking, he created many very effective formulas for treating tuberculosis and bone density problems.

Over 110 books were published on internal medicine in the nineteenth and early twentieth centuries. Some were comprehensive; others focussed on one or more specific diseases, such as stroke, tuberculosis, and stomach and intestinal diseases. The principle of contagious diseases had also been recognized since the early nineteenth century, and medical professionals were aware of the need to isolate patients from healthy people in these cases.

Eye, Ear, Nose, and Throat Specialties

The earliest references to ophthalmic diseases appear in works dating from the early Han Dynasty (c. 200 B.C.), although specialty texts were not written until centuries later. The great doctor Sun Si Miao of the Tang Dynasty (618–906) devoted an entire book to the study of ophthalmology. His work was called *Yin Hai Jing Wei* ("The Exhaustive and Comprehensive Survey of the Silver Sea" ["silver sea" is a name for the eye taken from Buddhist classics]). In it, Doctor Sun described eighty-one diseases of the eye, including numerous prescriptions and instructions for needling and other therapeutic techniques.

Medical formulas and many surgical therapies for removal of masses and repairing slashes to the eyeball developed during the next centuries. A book published in 752—*Wai Tai Mi Yao* ("Secret Techniques from the Master's Podium")—gives the first detailed description of cataract removal by needle.

By the late fourteenth century, many common ophthalmologic problems, such as reversion of eye slash, conjunctivitis, eye bleeding, cataract, and the diffuse pupil, were being treated with medicinal formulas and primitive surgical techniques.

Toward the end of the Ming Dynasty, in 1628, a medical text called *Yan Ke Da Quan* ("Most Complete Eye Book") appeared. This book is so complete that it is often referred to by modern students. It describes the "golden needle" method for removal of cataracts, including charms that should be wrapped around the golden needle before the operation, and illustrations of the needles used.

In 1644, an important work by Fu Ren Yu, *Shen Shi Yao Han* ("The Treasure for Vision"), summarized and updated the information in earlier texts. It described for the first time the theory that all internal organs are connected to the eyes via special meridians. Using many case studies for illustration, the author introduced methods for applying acupuncture and moxibustion techniques in ophthalmic practice, and how to treat cataracts using the "golden needle[2] separating technique"; 108 eye diseases were recorded, along with 300 medicinal formulas and illustrative charts. This text was so complete that it has been known ever since as the encyclopedia of ophthalmology.

Toward the end of the eighteenth century, Yang Wu wrote *Yan Ke Da Cheng* ("Great Success in Ophthalmology"), in which he discussed the theories of the influence of atmospheric phenomena on the eye, as well as the connection of human moods with diseases of the eye and the combination of eye diseases with other general diseases such as cough, dysentery, malaria, and so on.

Although later publications, especially during the nineteenth and early twentieth centuries, have added to the therapeutic and surgical techniques recommended for eye diseases and supplemented information on rare eye diseases and modern terminology, *Shen Shi Yao Han* remains a classic, well-respected text in this field, and is still consulted today.

Laryngology

The first specialty text on diagnosis and therapy for diseases of the mouth, teeth, tongue, lips, and larynx is Xue Ji's *Kou Ci Lei Yao* ("Essentials of the Mouth and Teeth") published in 1528. The content is simple, but it is the first specialty book in laryngology in Chinese medical history.

One of the best books on this subject, so well written and researched that it is still in use today, appeared in 1838. *Chong Lou Yu Shi* ("Folding, Building, and the Jade Key"), written by Zheng Mei Jian, began with a brief introduction to the anatomy and physiology of the throat and larynx, and went on to describe the differentiation, therapy, and prognosis of diseases of the throat and larynx—including the therapy and prognosis of diphtheria. A special section in this text instructs the doctor in the use of acupuncture and moxibustion for throat problems.

At the close of the nineteenth century, several deadly infectious diseases of the larynx were common, and many doctors dedicated themselves to laryngology research. Over a hundred books were published in this specialty field alone, with an additional fifty devoted to Bai Hou (diphtheria) and other infectious diseases of the larynx. It was considered correct to suggest the use of pungent and cool medicine first, then to use the bitter and cold medicine to clear heat, and lastly to use sweet and cold medicine to increase body fluids. Pungent and warm medicine was contraindicated for diphtheria. Many effective formulas and acupuncture prescriptions for treating the complications of diphtheria were also developed during this period of intensive research.

Notes

1. For more on this great physician, see chapter 4.
2. Gold was recognized as having antiseptic properties, which is why gold needles were used for cataract surgery.

9

Medicine for Women and Children

Gynecology and Obstetrics

The Tang Dynasty (618–906 A.D.), which saw the first organized push toward medical education, also seems to have been the first time doctors were encouraged to specialize.

The first account of a successful treatment for an obstetrical problem appears in a biography of the renowned doctor Hua Tuo (148–208 A.D.). His biography states that he attended the wife of a General Li in childbirth. During the delivery, one twin was born healthy and alive, while the other died and remained in the womb. Using acupuncture both to reduce the mother's pain and to induce the dead fetus, Hua Tuo removed it without harm to the mother.

The next reference to pregnancy and neonatal care appears during the Southern and Northern Dynasties (420–590) in the records of a doctor named Xu Zhi Cai. His theories were later recorded in detail by Sun Si Mao in the sixth century in his comprehensive text *Qian Jin Yao Fang* ("A Thousand Gold Necessary Formulas"). Among Xu Zhi Cai's recommendations, echoed by Doctor Sun, were diet and rest requirements for each month of pregnancy. Sun laid great stress upon the importance of good hygiene during pregnancy. Acupuncture was not recommended, but eighteen herbal formulas were provided for monthly fetal care; the purpose of these was for nourishing the blood, calming, and tonifying the Yin and kidneys in order to promote fetal growth and prevent miscarriages.

Doctor Sun also expanded the available knowledge about other gynecological problems and described the symptoms and treatments for twenty-two diseases related to menstruation, vaginal discharge, pregnancy, and delivery. The number of therapeutic formulas listed for Ob/Gyn problems totaled an impressive 557.

Toward the end of the Tang Dynasty (618–906), a doctor named Jiu Yin amassed the achievements and experiences of his predecessors, including folk formulas, and wrote *Jing Xiao Chan Bao* ("Treasured Techniques for Menstruation and Delivery"), which is the earliest medical text devoted entirely to gynecology and obstetrics. Unfortunately, only three volumes of this work survived. The first volume discusses problematic menstruation and vaginal discharge during pregnancy, and provides therapeutic formulas. The second volume discusses pregnancy and difficult delivery, and the third, various post-natal problems. The book prescribes three very effective formulas for morning sickness. It states precisely that there were two possible factors that would cause miscarriage: a sick mother or a malformed fetus. Several formulas were included to calm an overactive fetus, using such herbs as mugwort, angelica, and donkey gel. All the formulas recommended in this book are still in use today for these problems.

In the case of difficult delivery, both oral medication and surgical manipulation were recommended; these suggestions remain guiding principles to this day. The oral preparations included tonics and strengthening medicines to increase the mother's energy level.

After delivery, the author noted, the mother often suffers thirst and frequent urination; the pathological reasons given were loss of body fluids and blood, and damage to the urinary bladder during delivery. The appearance of a breast carbuncle after delivery was explained as follows: If newborns are not breast-fed, milk accumulates and ferments, causing the sore. The author prescribed a honey suppository for post-delivery constipation, and discouraged the use of purgatives. He suggested using vinegar fumes to revive patients from fainting spells.

During the Song and Yuan Dynasties (960–1368), as evidenced by several books that appeared at that time, the specialties of gynecology and obstetrics progressed rapidly. *Shi Chan Lun* ("Ten Topics on Baby Delivery") included the first record in history of a repositioning of a breach birth. Published in 1098, the book by Yang Zi Jian also described several techniques for assisting delivery, including transverse delivery, reverse delivery, and seated delivery, among others.

Less than fifty years later, a doctor named Yu Liu recorded a pill for inducing labor, the source of which was the brain of a rabbit. It has since been corroborated by modern medicine that a certain pituitary hormone available from rabbits can promote uterine contractions.

Perhaps the greatest contribution to gynecology and obstetrics during this period was made by Chen Zhi Ming (1190–1270) who wrote *Fu Ren Da Quan Liang Fang* ("General Health Formulas for Women"). Born in Jiang Xi Province, Chen carried on the family medical tradition for the third generation. His book, published in 1237, was the most comprehensive Ob/Gyn text of its time, covering menstruation, fertility, and miscellaneous gynecological diseases. It was pointed out, for example, that infertility could be caused by such factors as deficient Qi and blood, blood stasis,[1] and irregular menstruation with profuse discharge.

In obstetrics, Chen discussed five topics: stages of fetal growth, how to educate the fetus[2], how to ensure a safe pregnancy, complications during delivery, and post-delivery care for mother and child. Chen also discusses post-natal care, recommending several nursing procedures, and provided general suggestions for infant care, including infectious diseases.

From the Ming through the Qing Dynasties (1368–1912), hundreds of specialized texts on obstetrics and gynecology were published, among them new editions of earlier classics. Early in the eighteenth century, a book appeared that explained in simple language the three most important factors involved in the delivery procedure: Shun (sleep), Ren Tong (tolerance of pain), and Man Lin Pen (slow delivery). This book, called *Da Sheng Pian* ("Treatise on Taking Care of Life"), written by Ji Zai Ju Shi in 1715, became a basic introduction to general hygiene for women.

Advances in therapeutic techniques were introduced early in the nineteenth century by the renowned scholar and gynecologist Fu Qing Zhu. For vaginal discharge, infertility and hemorrhage, Fu's book (*Fu Qing Zhu Nu Ke*) offered extremely clear descriptions. His treatment for these problems emphasized tonifying the blood and Qi, and the spleen and stomach. This book holds a very important position in the history of Chinese medicine, because it clearly teaches that the spleen and stomach are the original sources for Qi (energy) and blood after birth.

Nu Ke Yao Lie ("Digest of Gynecology"), written by Pan Wei in 1877, is the most well-known gynecological text from this period. Pan Wei studied the classical literature, focusing his research and writing on regulating menstruation, calming the fetus, and prenatal and postpartum care. His chapter on regulating menstruation was especially thorough.

Pediatrics

Chinese medicine in pediatrics has its great advantage. Many very effective remedies are convenient and have no side effects. According to the existing records, many texts on pediatrics were already in publication by the Jin and Southern-Northern Dynasties (265–590), but most of them, unfortunately, have been lost. During the Tang Dynasty (618–906), which was generally a period of government support for medical education, a department of pediatrics was established in the National Health Administration. Five years of study was the minimum requirement for a doctor to be certified with a specialty in pediatrics. Infant care, including breast-feeding, had already been described in Doctor Sun Si Miao's comprehensive text *Qian Yin Yi Fang* ("A Thousand Essential Golden Formulas"), which appeared in the sixth century. The first medical text solely devoted to pediatrics, entitled *Lu Xin Jing* ("Treatise on the Fontanel"), was published sometime during the Sui and Tang Dynasties (590–906). This was the first book to describe how to use the wrist pulse diagnosis technique in babies.

Many common childhood diseases, such as convulsions, dysentery, and rash, were recorded in great detail, along with the appropriate principle and formula. For example, the author stated that bone-steaming syndrome (consumptive disease) with low-grade fever was caused by malnutrition and could be treated with tortoise shell. Tortoise shell was administered either by cooking it and drinking the broth, powdering the shell and eating it, or extracting and eating the gel.[3]

Pediatrics was not developed as an independent discipline until the Song Dynasty (although earlier medical texts did contain much information about treating children). The leading expert during this period was Qian Yi (1035–1117). Born in Shandong Province, Qian Yi devoted himself to pediatrics for forty years, amassing abundant clinical experience. He published nothing during his lifetime, but two years after his death, his students edited and published his work in three volumes called *Xiao Er yao Zheng Zhi Jue* ("Techniques of Pediatric

Medicine"), in which his principles on medicine for children were explained. All of the common childhood diseases were discussed with regard to diagnosis, differentiation, and therapy. The book included twenty-five case studies, herbal formulas used by the great doctor, and the physiology and pathology of disease. He systematically explained the stages of development in the five Zang organs (heart, liver, spleen, lung, and kidney) and the six Fu (small and large intestines, gall bladder, stomach, triple burner, and urinary bladder). He noted that disease can progress quickly due to excess at one time and deficiency at another. Detailed descriptions of symptoms were presented. As for treatment, Dr. Qian had advocated the use of Rou Rui (gentle and soft therapy), or making the choice of moderate therapy over extreme measures. He also emphasized that tonifying and reducing treatments should be used together on a child's delicate organs.

Based on these principles, Dr. Qian created the most effective medicinal formulas in pediatric history, some of which are still in use today. These include Cimicifuga rhizome and Pueraria root decoction for the initial eruption of chicken pox; the Dao Chi San for urinary tract infection; the Yi Gong San for poor digestion due to spleen and stomach Qi deficiency; and the Liu Wei Di Huang Wan formula for kidney yin deficiency.

Early in the thirteenth century, doctors were examining congenital diseases, especially noting the similarity between convulsions in adults and the neonatal convulsion syndrome caused by infection of the umbilicus. One author suggested use of a special iron for cutting the umbilical cord. The same author recorded a new technique of observing finger veins—instead of wrist—to diagnose disease in children younger than three years of age. While the first instance of this technique suggests using all ten fingers in the analysis, later work by a doctor named Liu Fang refined the technique by concentrating on the color and size of the vein in the index finger. This technique is still practiced by modern pediatricians in Traditional Chinese Medicine. Briefly, if the vein is visible primarily at the base of the finger (called Feng Guen, or the Wind Gate), the disease is in the early stages and can be easily cured. If the vein reaches to the first knuckle (Qi Guen, the Energy Gate), the disease is more severe. If the vein can be seen reaching to the third knuckle (Ming Guen, the Life Gate), the disease is in a dangerous condition.

The most important achievements in the field of pediatrics during the reign of the Ming and Qing Dynasties (1368–1912) may be summarized as follows:

Xue Kai (1372–?) emphasized the importance of mother's milk in determining the baby's health. He believed that disorders occurring during the breast-feeding period for babies are related to the mother's constitution, emotional status, and diseases. Therefore, he advocated treating the baby most effectively by treating the mother at the same time. His books included numerous case studies.

Wan Quan (1495–1580), whose grandfather and father were both accomplished pediatricians, studied and practiced pediatrics for over fifty years. He summarized his ancestors' and his own clinical experiences in ten medical texts.

Considering the child's delicate internal organs, his advice was to regulate mildly to balance the child's system, tonifying and reducing gently. Due to fact that Qi (energy) and the blood of children are not steady and strong, he believed that most children's cases could be cured by mild regulating therapy; strong therapy, he felt, should be avoided. Wan Quan described the pathogenic factors of acute and chronic convulsion in children, and he observed the complications after convulsions, such as paralysis and speech loss. Regarding malnutrition, he believed the main pathogenic source to be spleen and stomach, although he recognized that disorders in all organs can also cause malnutrition.

Over a hundred formulas for pediatric disease were recorded in his books. Yu Shu Dan, one of the most effective medicines still used in pediatrics (for convulsion, severe diarrhea, and vomiting) was first mentioned in this book, which also included many excellent prescriptions for nursing and child health preservation. His recommended technique for cutting the umbilical cord using burning scissors was an original sterilization technique.

In 1607, Wang Ken Tang claimed that childhood diseases are easy to treat, because children are not attacked by Qi Qing Liu Yu (seven emotional disturbances and six desires), and their organs are not abused by Ba Zhen Wu Wei (eight greasy/delicious food and five tastes). He believed that, after making a correct diagnosis, a quick response can be expected after applying medicine or relative therapy. This book was the first to record unblocking surgery for congenital obstruction of the anus. He suggested use of the Golden Knife[4] to open it, followed by application of Su He Xiang Wan (a very effective patent medicine) in the anus to induce the stool, thus saving the baby's life.

In 1750, Chen Fu Zheng described many external therapies for children, believing that because of their delicate and fragile organs, oral medicines should not be used unless absolutely necessary. His recommended therapies for children included pediatric massage, heat pad, herbal medicine patch, pricking with a needle, Gua Sha (stroking the child's spinal area with a silver coin or silver spoon to stimulate the important acupoints along the spine, thereby increasing the energy of the internal organs), and honey suppositories.

Many books about rash and skin lesions appeared during this period, including the first appearance of the disease name of "measles" and the principles for distinguishing measles from smallpox.

Other infectious diseases that demanded the constant attention of the pediatrician, such as chicken pox, were treated in several publications from the nineteenth century. Among them was a treatise solely on measles written by Zhang Xia Xi, who collected the clinical experiences of many renowned doctors on the pathogenesis, clinical manifestations, complications, treatment contraindications, and recommended therapy.

As mentioned above, medical massage for the treatment of children was first mentioned in the mid-eighteenth century. About a hundred years later, a complete text on massage manipulation for common pediatric diseases, including charts illustrating the points and manipulation techniques, appeared. In 1889, another treatise on medical massage, more comprehensive still, included diagnostic techniques for children, such as palpation of the chest and abdomen, a technique rarely mentioned elsewhere.

In China today, the primary medical modalities used on children are herbal treatments. Antibiotics are used as well, though only when absolutely necessary. Massage along the spinal column is still very popular, especially for poor digestion or other common chronic diseases.

Notes

1. As used in Traditional Chinese Medicine, the term "blood stasis" or "blood stagnation" refers not simply to the movement of blood through veins, but in a wider sense encompasses all the fluids and energy movements in the body. The theory holds that free-flowing energy in all forms is necessary for optimum health.

2. This term seems to have meant something similar to current theories about how to improve a baby's temperament and encourage growth while still in the womb, such as listening to good music, keeping the mother happy and feeding her good food, and so on.

3. Tortoise shell gel is also one of the preparations commonly prescribed for longevity.

4. This was similar to a modern scalpel, but was made of gold because of gold's antiseptic properties.

10
Anatomy, Surgery, and Trauma

Anatomy

Because of its connection to various ancient philosophies, Chinese medical theory seems to have an abstract nature, leading some scientists to assume that it is based on imagination rather than fact and to criticize the apparent neglect of the study of anatomy and organ and tissue structure. That this is an incorrect view of Chinese medical theory is borne out by the theory of viscera, bowel, and meridians/channels, which holds an important position in the Chinese medical system and is discussed in great detail in the *Nei Jing* (see chapter 1). This theory is important in the diagnosis and treatment of disease as well as forming the basis of the practice of acupuncture—one of the central treatment modalities of Traditional Chinese Medicine (see chapter 6).

Many people also become confused about anatomy and physiology in Chinese medicine due to improper translation of physiological concepts, which in turn is due to oversimplification of a very complex subject. In fact, the ancient Chinese are known to have been quite accurate in their anatomical observations.

One section of *Nei Jing* describes in great detail the physiological function and the general structure of the five Zang ("firm") organs (heart, liver, spleen, lung, and kidney) and six

Fu ("hollow") organs (small intestine, gall bladder, stomach, large intestine, bladder, and "triple burner" [san jiao]). The triple burner is a unique and controversial organ in Chinese medicine. Respiration, circulation, digestion, reproduction, immunity, and other processes are all based on the function of these internal organs. Dissections are recorded in the earliest medical texts, the *Nei Jing* and *Nan Jing*. In *Nei Jing*, the study of anatomy and dissection was advocated: "The body has skin and muscle. From outside, these can be measured. When a person dies, the body can be dissected and studied to evaluate the condition and size of the inner organs. The organs have a general size." In this section it was stated that the ratio of intestine to esophagus was 35:1, which is approximately equal to the 37:1 ratio known by modern anatomy. Blood circulation, not acknowledged by Western medicine until 1628 by William Harvey, was described in many parts of the *Nei Jing* at least fourteen hundred years earlier.

During the Han Dynasty (202 B.C.–220 A.D.), Wang Mang directed the National Medical Administration to utilize anatomical techniques for research, and the important text written by Sun Si Miao during the Tang Dynasty, *Qian Jin Yao Fang*, also contained references to studies of anatomy. During the Song Dynasty, when great strides were being taken in the subject, as well as in the art of drawing anatomical charts, two principal books were published. The charts contained therein were some of the earliest in world medicine.

The first was Ou Xi Fan (Charts of the Five Organs), which also included some pathological descriptions. For example, it was pointed out that under the lung are the heart, liver, gall bladder, and spleen. Under the stomach there are the small and large intestines, with the urinary bladder located to the side of the latter. Further, the text recorded two kidneys, one located under the right corner of the spleen and the other at the lower left. The observations concerning the liver, kidneys, heart, and intestines were so accurate that they could not have been made without an internal study of anatomy. Some of the views of pathology also were correct, such as "Meng Gan suffered from a cough; his lungs and gall bladder were black," or "Ou Quan had experienced eye problems as a child; there were white spots on his liver."

The second major book on anatomy was *Cun Zhen Tu*, written by Yang Jie. Its six charts portrayed major systems of the body: 1) the heart, including the entire cardiovascular system, 2) the diaphragm, including the penetrating blood vessel (the aorta) and esophagus, 3) the spleen and stomach, illustrating the digestive system, 4) the urinary system, 5) the life gate, intestine, and urinary bladder, and the reproductive system, and 6) the respiratory system.

Modern observations have verified the accuracy of most of the charts and explanations in this text. For hundreds of years afterward, authors quoted from *Cun Zhen Tu* when discussing anatomy.

During the Tang and Song periods (618–1279), anatomy made remarkable progress. But toward the end of the Song Dynasty, the philosophical theory known as Li Xue gained in popularity. Because one of its premises was that a person's body is inherited from his parents' bodies, it was thought that dissecting a body would desecrate the parents. As a result, anatomy and dissection were prohibited during this period. This political setback resulted in no progress in anatomy at least until the early part of the Qing dynasty (seventeenth century). There are no written records pertaining to the subject until some two hundred years later.

Early Forensic Medicine

The first text on forensic medicine was compiled by a commissioner of justice named Song Ci sometime during the years 1241–1253. It is divided into five volumes, the first of which discusses inquests, criminal abortion, infanticide, signs of death and human anatomy. The second covers murderous assaults, suicides, death by hanging, strangling, drowning, and burning. The third and fourth are concerned with poisoning and its antidotes, and the fifth contains instructions for the examination of the dead.

No post-mortems were performed at the time, and conclusions about the cause of death were made by external observation or by certain tests. Many of the tests seem to be fanciful, such as striking a blow on the rope of a hanging victim to determine, by the resulting vibration, whether the death was a murder or a suicide; or determining if two people were related by whether drops of blood from each run together or apart when dropped in water. Nevertheless, some conclusions were obviously based on keen observation—a particular talent of Chinese doctors throughout the ages. For example, if a body was found in the water, signs such as the abdomen being much distended would show that he or she must have been alive upon entering the water.

By the nineteenth century, doctors were again studying and publishing in the field of anatomy. One of the first books to appear was *Yi Lin Gai Cuo,* ("Correcting Mistakes in the Medical Field") by Wang Qing Ren (1768–1831) and published in 1830. Wang was born in Yu Tian, Hebei Province. His creed was: "To practice medicine and diagnosis, first of all one must know the anatomy and physiology." After years of practice and creative research, he corrected many mistakes about the internal organs that appeared in the standard medical texts of the day. He was able to study anatomy partly because of a custom of the time: families were forbidden to bury their dead children in the family tomb unless they had reached a certain age; there were designated places where families would discard the bodies of children younger than required for a proper burial. Wang Qing Ren encountered many such corpses. Because wild dogs had usually torn apart the bodies before Wang arrived, he was able to observe many aspects of the internal organs without actually cutting the bodies himself. Using this method he was able to observe and record the details of more than thirty corpses.

Wang Qing Ren was clearly an innovative and dedicated scientist. In spite of what must have been an overpoweringly bad odor, he observed and recorded the existence of such features as the aorta (Fu Zhu Dong Mai), the "largest vein vessel" (Shang Qiang jing Mai), pancreas, and diaphragm. His observation also led him to believe that the brain was the seat of memory, not the heart, as was commonly thought.

Surgery and Trauma

During the early years of the Han Dynasty (202 B.C.–220 A.D.), it was written in the *Huan Nan Zi*, "If there is a foreign object in the eye, but it does not affect sight, do not burn it; if there is an obstruction in the larynx which does not affect breathing, do not chisel it out." Passages such as these indicate that primitive surgical techniques were being developed contemporaneously with Greek and Roman doctors such as Galen in the West.

One of the First Surgeons
Hua Tuo, also known as Yuan Hua (145–208 A.D.), was born in Anhui Province. An outstanding medical doctor and scientist, he holds a very important position in Chinese medical history.
He refused to take orders from the imperial court (extremely dangerous behavior in a time when one's rulers were

considered to be on a par with God!) and insisted on practicing medicine among the common folk. He cured an innumerable number of patients and was respected and loved by them. In his later years, Hua Tuo was ordered to attend government officials. Cao Cao, the Emperor of Wei State during the period known as the Three Kingdoms, suffered from severe migraine headaches. Whereas all of the other physicians had failed, Hua Tuo used acupuncture and cured him. As a result, the emperor forced him to become his personal physician.

Using a pretext, Hua Tuo escaped to his home and refused to return. Furious, Cao Cao had him captured and ordered his execution. Just before his death, he offered his book to a custodian at the prison, urging him to preserve it by saying, "This book can cure people." But the jailer refused, saying that he was terrified at the prospect of being accused of having committed an offense. Hua Tuo therefore burned his book in a fit of rage at being unappreciated and took his knowledge with him to his death. What we today call the *Zhong Zang Jing* was not written by Hua Tuo but rather by someone else who used his name.

In addition to his expertise in many specialties such as internal medicine, gynecology, pediatrics, and acupuncture, Hua Tuo was well known as a surgeon. He invented the herbal anesthetic formula Ma Fei San, which he used on patients when he performed surgery. According to an account of Hua Tuo taken from *Hou Han Shu,* a historical record of the latter part of the Han Dynasty, "if the patient suffers from problems in the internal organs where medicines and needles cannot reach, Hua Tuo will let the patient drink the Ma Fei San with wine until he becomes drunk and unconscious. Hua Tuo will then open the patient's abdomen and back to remove the mass. Should the problem be in the stomach and intestines, Hua Tuo will cut the intestine, wash it to remove the diseased part, suture it, and cover the wound area with a very effective ointment. The healing period for the wound is approximately four or five days; one month later the patient can expect complete recovery."

A story is told of a time when Hua Tuo was treating the emperor Cao Cao for severe headaches. Based on his observation of the emperor's symptoms, Hua Tuo diagnosed a brain tumor, and offered to use his surgical skills to open the emperor's skull and remove the tumor. Cao Cao refused, however, fearing a plot to assassinate him, and would accept only acupuncture treatment for his pain. Hua Tuo complied, but the emperor's headaches eventually worsened and he died, most probably from the tumor that Hua Tuo has diagnosed.

From the Jin Dynasty (265–420 A.D.), some records describe how to repair a harelip. During the Sui and Tang Dynasties (590–906), dental and optical surgery developed to a moderate extent. During the Tang Dynasty, the use of combined silver, lead, and mercury was introduced for tooth fillings.

Between 475 and 502 A.D., Gong Qing Xuan of the state of South Qi wrote what is thought to be the first book that primarily addressed surgery: the *Liu Jue Zi Gui Yi Fang* (*Formulas from fairies through Liu Jue Zi*). Subjects included traumatic injuries incurred in war, carbuncles, cellulitis, lymphoma, eczema, psoriasis, as well as many other dermatological problems. Among other subjects, this book also discussed 140 herbal prescriptions for both internal and external use.

For cases of traumatic injury, Gong prescribed treatments for halting bleeding and for pain relief. Methods for tranquilization, detoxification, and applying stringents were described, as well as new kinds of ointment and patch medical remedies, such as a mixture of mercury, rhubarb, and coptis root for the treatment of carbuncles.

At this time, the therapeutic principles, such as herbal medicines, that were known to help with internal medicine had not been transferred to the surgical sciences. However, the author, while discussing the oral administration of herbal medicines, emphasized the necessity for differentiation of syndromes. His ideas formed the basis for three therapeutic principles to be followed in treating surgical diseases. For example, for a carbuncle, he suggested to first differentiate the cause of the pus (hot, cold, etc.), then drain it with a cauterized needle. The third principle concerned the essential component of wound healing, which was thinning of the blood.

The introduction with this book of this principle of improving the circulation of the blood greatly improved the effectiveness of treating diseases surgically, because it was now recognized that proper circulation was necessary for wound healing. This idea was further improved upon in the Qing Dynasty (1644–1912 A.D.) by the renowned doctor Weng Qing Ren, who observed that the blood stagnates in the organs of dead people, and from his observations devised the theory of blood stasis, or poor circulation of the body fluids, to explain the cause of many diseases. This theory is still a guiding principle today for doctors in how to treat various chronic diseases.

During the Sui and Tang Dynasties, serious attention was paid to carbuncles, cellulitis, and traumatic injury. Both the *Qian Jin Yao Fang* and the *Zhu Bing Yuan Hou Lun* contributed greatly to this research. For example, how to distinguish a carbuncle from another problem was recorded, as well as special formulas for treating fistula. *Zhu Bing Yuan Hou Lun,* in addition, described techniques for resection of the intestines, sealing blood vessels, and removing extraneous material from the injured area.

Cao Yuan Fang was a doctor who practiced in about 600 A.D. His book (written in collaboration with other doctors) *Zhu Bing Yuan Hou Lun* ("Etyiology and Manifestation of Many Diseases") is one of the classics of symptom description (see chapter 1). This comprehensive treatise also discusses some surgical topics, such as techniques to induce abortion, for intestine reconnection, and for some dental surgery. Unfortunately, the author included no detailed case studies.

Also discussing carbuncles and abscesses (the most common types of surgical problems) was *Wei Ji Bao Shu* (Treasure Book for Hygiene and Health), written by an unknown author early in the twelfth century. Therapeutic principles were established in this text, such as promoting muscle growth, testing and draining pus, injection of medicines, moxibustion treatment for abscesses, and others. The author recommended forty herbal formulas for surgical diseases.

This book also focused on cancer for the first time in written history. Skin masses, cellulitis, and internal organ masses were some of the other topics. In its discussion of breast cancer, for example, *Wei Ji Bao Shu* observed that this disease often attacks women over forty and that the tumor metastasizes and, after three years, causes the patient's death. His conclusions have since been corroborated by modern medicine.

Li Xun's *Ji Yan Bei Zu Fang*, written in 1196, differentiated between exterior and interior abscesses, noting that on the exterior of the body, they are easily treatable despite fever, swelling, and pain. However, treatment of an abscess inside of an organ, even without other clinical manifestations, is difficult.

In the year 1264, further knowledge about malignancies was forthcoming when Yang Shi Ying wrote *Ren Zai Zhi Zi Fang*. Following is his description of a malignant tumor: "uneven surface, like rocks and caves; granula folds [nodule is hard and unmoving], the toxin root can penetrate deep in the body."

In 1263, Chen Zhi Ming wrote the *Wai Ke Jing Yao*, a three-volume work in which he emphasized the importance of differentiating among syndromes when treating surgical diseases. During this period, most doctors believed that abcesses and boils were the result of heat toxin. Chen, however, felt that many types of pathogenic mechanisms besides toxic heat could cause surgical diseases. He maintained that all prescriptions should differentiate the deficiency or excess of Zang Fu organs and channels since not all surgical diseases were caused by the heat toxin, and that overuse of cold and detoxifying medicine could delay recovery. This line of thinking greatly contributed to the use of oral medicine as a treatment of surgical disease, in order to avoid the dangers of surgery.

No work specifically on the subject of traumatology appeared until *Wai Ke Jing Yao* (1266 A.D.) written by Chen Zhi Ming. This work symbolized the emergence of surgery and traumatology as legitimate specialties. Due to the many wars that punctuated Chinese history to this point, battlefield injuries had allowed Chinese surgeons many opportunities to experiment with different treatments.

Another important surgical text during this period, the six-volume *Ji Jiu Xian Fang*, introduced treatment for carbuncles, abscesses, eye diseases, hemorrhoids, skin lesions, and other conditions. The author included many herbal formulas appropriate for use by internists, gynecologists, and pediatricians.

At that time, carbuncles and abscesses were thought to be the products of an internal heat syndrome. The two main therapeutic principles were either to dissolve it or to increase body resistance to flush out the toxin. They were first recorded in *Tai Ping Sheng Hui Fang*. ("Formulas for Peace and Charity") (982–992) by Wang Huai Yin. *Sheng Ji Zong Lu* ("Comprehensive Collection of Surviving Techniques"), a government publication appearing about 1111–1117, advocated orally administered medicine together with surgery to treat carbuncle. The major surgical tools included knives, needles, hooks, clips, and other instruments.

Summarizing advances in surgery in the period between the Song and Yuan Dynasties, *Wai Ke Jing Yi* encompassed two volumes and was written by Qi De Zhi in 1335. The first volume discussed miscellaneous surgical diseases, such as boils, carbuncles, and abscesses. The second volume listed 145 formulas for herbal medicines in varied dosage forms. Many new techniques were suggested, especially for removal of pus, such as how to remove pain with moxibustion, and the use of medicinal pastes and patches.

During the Yuan Dynasty, several books on surgery and trauma addressed the subject of orthopedics as well. Two books that appeared in the first half of the fourteenth century devoted many pages to bone fracture and joint dislocation. The treatment techniques were quite sophisticated, including several recommendations for dislocated joints, one of which emphasized traction. Another mode of treatment was to reset the fractured bone and immobilize the joint by means of bamboo wood splints instead of gypsum casts (as are used today), although gypsum casts seem to have been in use at that time as well.

For suturing, surgeons used a curled needle and sutures made of silk or white mulberry bark. Several common anesthesias included those prepared from aconite root and Metl flower.

During the sixteenth century, surgeons increased their understanding of what caused surgical disease, invented or improved on existing surgical tools, and published many books on the subject. Some of these included case studies for the first time such as *Zheng Ti Lei Yao* written by Dr. Xue Ji in 1529. It described nineteen ways to manipulate dislocated joints and other case studies.

The subject of cancer appears again in a work called *Wai Ke Shu Yao*, published in 1571 and written by Xue Ji. His book dealt with the treatment of different types of masses and lumps in both skin and organs. The author classified all masses into thirty categories, a few of which are Jin (tendon) tumor, blood tumor, Rou (muscle) tumor, Qi tumor (lymphoma), and bone tumor.

An important text that covered surgery, traumatology, and orthopedics was called *Yang Yi Zheng Zhi Zhun Sheng* ("Standard Therapy for Surgical Diseases"). This book, written by

Wang Ken Tang, was published in 1608. Wang suggested that the orthopedics doctor should be well equipped with anatomical knowledge. He introduced many surgical techniques, some recorded for the first time. These included brachia ligament surgery and ear floppy plastic surgery, recording the entire procedures step by step. This is the first appearance of plastic surgery used both cosmetically and therapeutically. There is a description of how to repair a harelip as well as how to "pin" ears back. Following is a description for throat repair: "If the patient's throat has been cut, suture the inside membrane of the throat (brachia). Then the outside skin. Seal with herbal ointments to promote healing and stop the bleeding. Change the medicines daily. To treat patient with ear injury or ear that has fallen off, use powders that promote healing for sticking the ear in right position. Then, using the goose feather or small bamboo splint, fix it according to damage. Remember to check both ear symmetry."

For the traumatological injury of head, neck, scapular bone, chest, hip, and spine, he suggested emergency and resuscitation techniques. For the treatment of masses, he suggested that if the mass is movable, surgery can be used to remove the mass. If the mass is unmovable and fixed, it is better not to interfere with surgery.

During this period, acute appendicitis was well recognized. In *Yi Xue Zheng Zhuan* (Biography in Medical Format), written in 1500 by Dr. Yu Tuan (1438–1517), it was described thus: "patient has a fever similar in appearance to malaria, and there is a painful, palpable mass in the right side of the lower abdomen which limits the extension of the right leg, these are signs of Chang Yong (intestinal abscess)."

Wai Ke Zheng Zong ("Original Ancestor of Surgery") was published in 1617 and written by Chen Shi Gong (1555–1636). Chen dedicated his career to the subjects of surgery and traumatology, and *Wai Ke Zheng Zong* summarized the essence of his clinical experiences during forty years of practice. According to his theory, a disease that occurred inside the body may not necessarily extend to the outside, but a disease occurring outside the body must be rooted inside. When dealing with surgical problems, he recommended harmonizing the spleen and stomach using the therapeutic principles of Tuo (elevating) and Bu (tonifying) to speed the healing process. His book included many charts on the various diseases.

For the abscess, he advocated drawing the toxin out of the body by using a knife and needle to open the abscess and drain the poison out, or the use of strong medicine to erode the dead tissue. He also designed a special surgical tool for removing a mass from the nostril. For the treatment of hemorrhoids, he invented some brilliant surgical techniques, such as shrinking the hemorrhoid by tying off with threads. Wang's book also dealt with dermatological problems in detail and was the first to record a malignant lymph tumor in the neck, vividly describing its clinical manifestations. He created two formulas for this malignant tumor, which are still being used today. He did not claim that these formulas could cure the tumor, but they effectively relieved suffering and improved the patient's quality of life. His book also includes a correct description and prognosis for breast cancer.

Another text that addressed cancer during this period was *Wai Ke Da Cheng* ("Great Achievements in Surgery"), written by Qi Kun, who served as president of the Royal Health Administration during the early Qing Dynasty (1644–1912). Qi discussed four types of cancer that he recognized as incurable: Shi Rong (lymph tumor in neck area), She Gan (tongue cancer), Ru Yan (breast cancer), and Shen Yan (kidney cancer). His book introduced the diagnosis of common surgical diseases and the popular medicinal formulas related to them. For example, to treat an abscess with eruption of pus, he recommended soaking gauze with Xuan Zhu Gao, a kind of medicinal ointment, and inserting the gauze into the abscess to encourage drainage. This technique is still in use.

During the early eighteenth century, Wang Wei De distilled the clinical experiences of four generations of doctors in his family in *Wai Ke Zheng Zhi Quan Sheng Ji* ("Comprehensive Surviving Therapeutic Techniques for Surgical Diseases"), written in 1740. This important book classified surgical diseases into two categories: Yin and Yang, for example, Yong (abscess) belongs to the Yang syndrome; cellulitis belongs to the Yin syndrome. The author put more emphasis on tonifying the Qi and blood to promote the blood circulation with the warm medicine, disliking the clearing fire treatment with cold and cool medicine. He created many effective medicinal formulas, two of which, Xi Huang Wan and Xiao Jin Dan, are still considered the best medicine to prescribe for breast and liver cancer. A shortcoming of his book and theory was the refusal by the author to use the knife; he claimed that any disease could be cured by oral medicines alone.

Ma Pei Zhi came from a family that had been practicing medicine for three generations in the nineteenth century. They were especially well known for their knowledge about surgical and traumatological diseases. In treating surgical disease, Ma Pei Zhi emphasized differentiation of syndromes. He compiled his experience in surgical tools and formulas into a book entitled *Wai Ke Chuan Xin Lu* ("Successive Recordings of Surgery"—1892), but he is probably best known for his commentary and correction of the *Wai Ke Quan Sheng Ji,* which was considered a very valuable contribution by Chinese surgeons.

The doctor best known for skill in external medicine was Wu Shang Xian (1806–1886). With knowledge gleaned from his family's clinical experience in external medicine, he collected many old proven folk formulas and combined those with his own clinical experience to write *Li Yue Pian Wen* ("Poem of Disposing Surgical Diseases"—1864). For every disease, he combined the prescription of medicinal patches with specific techniques for their use, such as Dian (spotting), Chu (sneezing), Cha (rubbing), Yun (warm soothing), Luo (burning), Chan (mixing), and Fu (moist heating pad). This is a very comprehensive summarization for traditional external medicine. Medicinal patches continue to be a very popular dosage form.

One miraculously successful orthopedics doctor was Jiang Kao Qing, who wrote in his 1840 text on bone fractures: "When treating a bone fracture where parts of the bone have penetrated the muscle, one portion of anesthesia medicine Number Twelve should be administered to the patient. The wound area should then be cut open and the bone fragments removed and rearranged." If the bone was crushed beyond use, he replaced it with another bone. The use of oral anesthesia and the description of the bone transplant technique both indicated that orthopedics surgery was very advanced at this time.

In dealing with bone fractures today, Chinese medicine uses a combination of Western and Chinese therapies. X rays are used to determine the extent of the damage and the procedure for setting the fracture. Then a system of Chinese splints is used rather than the heavy plaster casts found in the West, which often immobilize not only the area of the fracture but also the points above and below the break. The splints allow the knitting process of the fracture to take place without creating the stiffness in the nearby joints or the muscle wastage a cast would cause, and speed up overall rehabilitation.

Surgical techniques in the late nineteenth and early twentieth centuries declined somewhat due to lack of advancement in the natural sciences and the corresponding growth of those disciplines in Western medicine. However, many herbal preparations are still used in combination with Western-type surgeries, such as ointments applied via patches to promote wound healing or to remove dead tissue.

An interesting footnote to surgical history is the advent of the refined techniques of microsurgery. Although the technology for this advanced form of surgery originated in the West, it was a Chinese doctor, Chen Zhong Wei, who first perfected the technique in 1965.

IV
Professional Standards

11
A Note on Medical Ethics

The Hippocratic oath, which to this day is solemnly repeated by new physicians in the West, is a testament to the dedication and seriousness with which doctors have regarded their profession since earliest times. In China, such dedication was often taken for granted until the Tang Dynasty, when an oath similar to that of Hippocrates was circulated. It is possible that physicians felt they simply did not need such an oath prior to that time. Perhaps this attitude sprang from the reverence in which the healing arts were held, viewed as they were as direct gifts from the gods revealed to humankind through the hands of the divinely appointed rulers—the three "celestial emperors" in particular—who transmitted all the skills and knowledge necessary for building a great civilization. Sometime during the Tang Dynasty (618–906 A.D.), a code for doctors was created, which has persisted to this day in spirit, although it is not part of the ritual of medical training in China as the Hippocratic oath is in the West.

The Hippocratic Oath

I swear by Apollo the healer, by Asclepias, by Hygeia, by Panacea and by all the gods and goddesses, making them my witness, that I will carry out, according to my ability and my judgment, this oath and this indenture. To hold my teacher in this art equal to my own parents; to make him partner to my livelihood; when he is in need of money to share mine with him; to consider his family as my own brothers and to teach them this art, if they want to learn it, without fee or indenture; to impart precept, oral instruction, and all other instruction to my own sons, the sons of my teacher, and to indentured pupils who have taken the physician's oath, but to nobody else.

I will use treatment to help the sick according to my ability and judgment, but never with a view to injury and wrongdoing. Neither will I administer a poison to anybody when asked to do so, nor will I suggest such a coarse. Similarly I will not give a woman a pessary to cause abortion. But I will keep pure and holy both my life and my art. I will not use the knife, not even, verily, on sufferers from stone, but will place to such as are craftsmen therein.

Into whatever houses I enter, I will enter to help the sick and I will abstain from all intentional wrong-doing and harm, especially from abusing the bodies of man or woman, bond or free. And whatsoever I shall see or hear in the course of my profession, as well as outside my profession in my intercourse with men, it if be what should not be published abroad, I will never divulge, holding such things to be holy secrets. Now if I carry out this oath, and break it not, may I gain forever reputation among all men for my life and for my art; but if I transgress it and forswear myself, may the opposite befall me.

The Chinese version of this oath, which appeared sometime during the Tang Dynasty, reads as follows:

If you would be a great doctor.
 . . . when you begin treatment, you should calm your mind so you can attend to your patient without any distraction. With great charity of heart, resolve to save your patient.

If you would be a great doctor,
 . . . do not consider whether your patient is rich or poor, from the upper or lower class, old or young, stupid or intelligent,

beautiful or ugly, an enemy or a friend, a citizen or a foreigner. All patients are equal before you; treat them all as you would your dearest friend or a member of your family.

If you would be a great doctor,
  ... do not put anything above the care of your patient—not your reputation, nor personal gain, nor any other affairs. Look to your patient's suffering as if it were your own suffering, with the greatest sympathy and attention. You may be called upon to travel long distances or endure hunger and fatigue in order to save your patient. You must do all this without complaint, pretention, or self-promotion.

If you would be a great doctor,
  ... do not be tempted by beautiful treasures in the home of your patient, or lovely music, or delicious food, or fragrant wine. Do not gossip or joke about others, and never speak ill of another doctor. When your patient is cured, do not boast about it and puff yourself up.

If you would be a great doctor, you must observe all these rules. If you do not, you are certainly a devil and a thief of life itself. These are the warnings for those who would become doctors.

Exemplary of this attitude of conscientious medicine is the renowned doctor of the Tang Dynasty, Sun Si Miao (581–682 A.D.), who made many contributions to Chinese medicine (see chapter 5). Perhaps most importantly, Sun greatly emphasized medical ethics, believing that it is a doctor's responsibility to treat all patients fairly and seriously, whether they be rich or poor, old or young. He regarded traditional medicine as a precious heritage and society's solemn duty to develop that heritage.

12
Medical Standards and the Education of Physicians

According to historical records dating from the Tang Dynasty, many states in China had, by 443 A.D., established systems for primary medical education. The Northern Wei State assigned titles to doctors such as Tai Yi Bo Shi ("Professor of Medicine"), Tai Yi ("Great Doctor"), and so on. During the Sui Dynasty (590–618), the government took an active part in training physicians when it established the National Health Administration. This agency was staffed by a chief pharmacist, a doctor, a gardener of herbal medicine, a professor and assistant professor of medicine, a massage instructor, and others.

During the Tang Dynasty (618–906), medical education reached an organizational peak. In the year 624, the Tang government established its own National Health Administration[1] composed of four departments: Administration, Medical Education, Pharmacy, and Clinical. The agency was headed by a man whose position was equal in power to that of the national premier. Altogether, his staff numbered about 340.

The medical education department contained four divisions: Internal Medicine (staff of 164), Acupuncture/Moxibustion (staff of fifty-two), Massage (staff of thirty-six), and Connotation[2] (staff of twenty-one). Medical students in each department began their training by reading and studying the medical classics *Su Wei* ("Plain Questions"), *Shen Nong Ben*

Cao Jing ("Shen Nong Pharmacopoeia"), *Mai Jing* ("Pulse Diagnosis"), and *Zhen Jiu Jia Yi Jing* ("ABCs of Acupuncture"). Following this general study, the students moved into specializations. Seven years of study were required for a specialist in internal medicine, five for pediatrics or traumatologists, and four for ophthalmologists and otorhinolaryngologists. The students were evaluated by means of examinations, and those who failed regularly were dropped from the program after nine years.

In addition to the National Health Administration, many local, private organizations devoted themselves to medical education and management. However, because the government's education program was situated in the capital city, and travel from far provinces unusual for most people, the most likely way for a doctor to be trained was to apprentice to another doctor in or outside his family. It was quite common for the medical profession to be handed down from father to son, each generation building on the accomplishments of the preceding one.

Medical Education and Regulation

During the Sony Dynasty (960–1279), another long-enduring administration, the new government again established its own National Health Administration. But this time the agency's mandates were extended to separate medical regulation from medical education, assign doctors to the areas of the country where they were most needed, and to assume responsibility for the prevention of epidemics.

At one time, during the year 1112, the agency's staff of physicians had increased to an all-time high of 1,096. To serve in the agency, a person was required to be at least forty years old and to pass a series of difficult exams. (After 1188, the agency included so-called folk doctors—those without an academic background, who practiced in the remote regions of the country—in its lists as well as those who could boast more formal training.) Doctors earned various ranks and titles according to their exam scores and technical skill. The best doctors were rewarded by being assigned to serve in the National Health Administration situated in the capital; others were assigned to be doctors and professors in other regions.

Since this system resulted in an uneven distribution of doctors between the central and remote areas, it became necessary to base assignments upon specialty. Therefore, in the year 1113, the agency created the following eight categories of medical specialties: general practitioner, internist, obstetrician, ophthalmologist, acupuncturist, dermatologist, dentist, and surgeon.

In addition to the government-run NHA, many private organizations sprang up to provide health care. For example, written histories of the period recount that, in the years between 1102 and 1249, various agencies dispensed health services to the poor, cared for indigent patients, served the needs of travelers seeking medical care, provided for the needs of the elderly, and cared for abandoned babies.

When the Song Dynasty undertook professional regulation of doctors, it established standard exams to cull out the unworthy, as well as continuing-education requirements to keep doctors current on advances in medicine. Furthermore, it instituted laws governing medical practice and recognized the increased need for medical ethics and liability. If a decision was handed down that a doctor had acted unscrupulously to gain financial advantage, he was punished with jail term similar to what a robber would receive, as well as having his medical license suspended. Laws like these greatly enhanced the image of the medical professions as well as improving efficacy and safety.

Medical education during the Song eventually reached a very high level. Early in the Song Dynasty, instructors were mandated to teach *Plain Questions* and *Nan Jing* with little variation. In 1061, the Royal Medical Administration, with a current student body of 120, enlarged its curriculum, adding the pharmacopoeia *Shen Nong Ben Cao Jing* to its list of required study materials. The medical school staff gained in reputation because, for the first time in a Chinese medical school, each department was headed by a professor who was required to be a physician of renown.

The 300 students who registered for the school, which began with the spring semester, were divided into three classes according to admission test scores: forty were assigned to the highest level, fifty to the intermediate, and 200 to the lowest. One private exam was held monthly, and a public one held yearly. Students earned points based on their attitude and manner as well as their knowledge and technique. Students practiced their techniques by treating members of the military, under supervision; their scores were computed according to the effectiveness of their treatments. Top-scoring students earned the chance to be promoted to the highest class. It is this examination process that is one of the major contributions of this time period.

During the year 1078 to 1085, the 300 medical students were divided into nine disciplines: 120 general practitioners, eighty neurologists, twenty internists, twenty orthopedists, ten obstetricians, twenty ophthalmologists, ten dental and throat doctors, ten acupuncturists, and ten traumatologists.

The Song Dynasty came at a time when China was still divided into several distinct states, each with its own rulers and traditions. It wasn't until the beginning of the Yuan Dynasty, in 1260, that China became unified into one country.[3] Because of this continuing social unrest, progress in medical education remained localized and moved at a slow pace until the early years of the Yuan. Nevertheless, the advances made during the Song showed significant improvement over those of the Tang.

During the Ming Dynasty (1368–1644), clinical specialties became more pronounced. The national health agency classified medicine into thirteen departments: internal medicine, infectious diseases, gynecology and obstetrics, pediatrics, dentistry, larynx and throat, ophthalmology, dermatology, orthopedics, traumatology, acupuncture and moxibustion, massage, and prayer. The classification for infectious diseases reflected the newest discoveries about pathogens. This is the first time that dentistry and throat specialties were separated, as were orthopedics and traumatology. This is also the first time we see massage as an independent specialty.

During the Ming and Qing Dynasties, medical education was governed by a national health agency as before, but, also as before, most doctors still relied on informal education and apprenticeship within families. In the Ming Dynasty, officials sought to formalize this training and encourage students to apply to the Royal Health Administration for their training. For this reason, the agency selected many of its students from among the children of doctors who had also served in this organization. At the same time, some students were recommended to the school from rural areas.

The students were assigned to different majors and specialties. Their textbooks included all the major classics, plus additional books on specialty medicine. Each student had to take four examinations per year, one in each season, and a major examination every three years. The examinations included both written tests and oral defense. Test scores were graded in three levels, the lowest of which represented failure. Students had one chance to retake the test; if they failed a second time, they were dropped from the program.

Just as the Ming Dynasty before it, the Qing government adopted measures to revive the economy. But history repeated itself, and a corrupt, inept regime sapped the strength of the country. Foreign imperialists invaded China in 1840, and the opium wars broke out. Thus the Ming-Qing era ended with China in a state somewhere between feudalism and capitalism, partially independent and partially colonized by foreign powers.

All this social and political unrest effectively stifled medical research and advances in education for decades. Not until the mid-twentieth century would medical education know the freedom and acceptance it had gained in the years of the Song and Yuan Dynasties.

The Dark Era for Chinese Medicine

In the early part of 1914, China was under the domination of the North Group Military Government. Wang Da Xie, the administrator of the educational department, wanted to reduce the use of traditional Chinese medicine. His policy naturally drew extensive criticism and opposition from professionals in the Chinese medical field. Doctors in every province organized "Chinese Medicine Rescue Petition Teams." Wang Da Xie's policy was finally withdrawn, but the national spiritual deficiency that had left an opening for such a policy remained. In 1925, an application by the National Education Association that appealed for the addition of Chinese medical courses to the required curriculum and for the establishment of the Department of Chinese Medicine in medical universities was refused by the Guoming Dang (National Party) government.

The activities designed to destroy Chinese medicine reached their peak in February 1929, when the first Central Hygiene Committee Conference was held by the government. Yu Yan was a doctor who had studied Western medicine in Japan and returned to China in 1916. Deeply prejudiced against Chinese medicine, about which he knew very little, he wrote two books attacking its precepts. At the conference, Yu Yan suggested that the old ways of medicine should be demolished. He said, "The theory of our national medicine is filled with ridiculous things. There is no way to keep that . . . if we want to protect the treasure of our nationality." He criticized even acupuncture and moxibustion as superstitious practices.

Yu's reasons for such a virulent attack on Chinese medicine included the following points:

1. The basic theory of Chinese medicine is based on the imagination.
2. Chinese pulse diagnosis is based on superstition and is fradulent.
3. Chinese medicine cannot prevent epidemic plague.
4. The pathogenesis theory obstructs the progress of science.

Yu Yan further suggested these concrete steps in order to abolish Chinese medicine completely:

1. To register all traditional Chinese medical doctors by the end of 1930.
2. To build a training center for traditional Chinese medical doctors, designed to educate them in Western medicine. After this training, doctors would receive a certificate, without which they could not practice medicine.
3. Traditional Chinese medical doctors with twenty years of practical experience could continue to practice. But that practice would be limited. They could not diagnose or treat infectious diseases or issue death certificates. This special license was limited in duration to fifteen years.
4. To prohibit the appearance of traditional Chinese medical knowledge in any public medium.

5. To close Traditional Chinese medical schools.

The subsequent approval of Yu's suggestions by the conference triggered furious reactions in the Chinese medical field. On March 17, 1929, the National Conference of the Chinese Medical Association was held in Shanghai. One hundred thirty-two organizations from fifteen provinces together petitioned the central government to cancel Yu's proposal. Due to the strength of the objections, the government did agree to cancel this proposal, but many restrictive regulations were put into place.

In 1933, Wang Jing Wei, vice president of the Guoming Dang government, drafted a "Management Proposal for Chinese Medicine," which advocated eliminating the practice of Traditional Chinese Medicine completely, and in the meantime placed even more limitations on its practice. In 1946, the Department of Education eliminated the Shanghai College of Traditional Chinese Medicine and the New China Medical School. The excuse given was the poor equipment in both schools. Twenty Chinese medical schools in Guangdong Province were reduced to only one, the Guangdong Chinese Medicine Specific School, by 1947.

Although the number of practitioners of Traditional Chinese Medicine dwindled during this period, it was impossible to abolish Chinese medicine completely. Its truly effective therapeutic results could not be denied, and it continued to earn support as the treatment modality of choice by most of the Chinese people.

The Building of Chinese Medical Schools, Associations, and the Publishing of the Journals of Chinese Medicine

Under the pressure of the decreasing availability of Chinese medicine brought about by the actions of a reactionary government, many noteworthy doctors dedicated themselves to protecting this precious medical system. Their contributions included building many Chinese medical schools, editing the traditional textbooks used to study the classic books such as the *Nei Jung* and other specialty medical textbooks.

These new medical schools educated large numbers of Chinese physicians, who became the majority of professional doctors continuing the development of Chinese medicine after 1949. But because these schools were private, they faced many problems, including lack of funds, poor equipment, and lack of teachers. This hampered the development of Chinese medicine and reflected poorly on the policies of the government.

Many professional associations also sprang up during this time in response to the drive to protect Traditional Chinese Medicine. The earliest was created in June 1906, in Shanghai. In 1912, a new organization was formed, that eventually grew to forty branches and over six thousand members. In 1913, the National Chinese Medical Association was created in Shanghai and Beijing, and in 1929, the National Chinese Physician Association appeared. In 1910 the first organization to promote the combination of Western medicine and Chinese medicine was formed. And in 1931, the earliest research organization for acupuncture and moxibustion was created.

Doctors also saw the establishment of many professional journals on both Chinese medicine and the combination of Chinese and Western theories. By 1949, more than four hundred journals were in circulation. The journals suffered from the same financial difficulties as the Chinese medical schools, and most did not last very long. Even so, these journals helped greatly to educate people about Chinese medicine and to promote communication among medical professionals. It also symbolized the continuous progress of Chinese medicine in its later stages of development.

Medical Education in the Modern Era

Due to the corruption of the late Qing Dynasty, the unstable social environment of the pre-republic stage as described above, and the Japanese invasion during World War II, the development of medical education slowed greatly. But with the importation of Western medicine into China in the late nineteenth century, the Qing government and foreign doctors together began to build medical schools to teach Western medicine.

According to a report by the Chinese Medical Association and the National Health Administration, at the end of World War II, 13,000 students had graduated from medical school and over 10,000 nurses and obstetrics assistants had received professional training. These people became the backbone of medicine and health care in China, and due to their contribution, it became possible for modern medicine to develop and grow quickly in China. But these medical professionals were far fewer than were needed to care for the huge population of old China.

In 1949, the Ministry of National Health and Hygiene (MNH) was created to oversee medical training and policy; it included a division devoted solely to Traditional Chinese Medicine. Until 1985, this division operated as an independent ministry to serve Traditional Chinese Medicine.

During the next decades, China survived many political movements, including the largest, known as the Great Leap Forward in 1958, and the full-scale eruption of the Great Proletarian Cultural Revolution, which lasted for ten years (1966–1976). Both movements had a devastating effect on China's economy and culture.

Mao Ze Dong and his premier, Zhou En Lai, were both believers in, and advocates of Chinese culture and Traditional

Chinese Medicine. Each had a personal doctor trained in Traditional Chinese Medicine. During this time (1950–1965), the economic condition of New China was very poor, due for the most part to the war with Japan (1937–1945) and the civil war that followed. Modern Western medical doctors were far away from those who needed treatment; even worse, most medications had to be imported. Most people could not afford that type of health care. All of these factors prompted the government to advocate the use of Chinese medicine as the major health-care modality and to support the education of Traditional Chinese Medicine practitioners.

Supplying doctors of TCM to satisfy the current need was the first priority of the government, which began by building "Combination Clinics" in most urban areas to attract and organize experienced Chinese medical doctors and encourage them to practice together. The next step was to gradually transfer these doctors to a larger scale health-care provider/organization—the hospital—and to prepare and select the best doctors for administrating and staffing medical schools.

In 1950, four Chinese medical schools were built: Beijing University of TCM, Shanghai College of TCM, Guangzhou College of TCM, and Chengdu College of TCM. Within five years, most provinces had their own Chinese medical school. All of these medical schools were public schools supported by the national and local governments. Students were selected by strict examination. The original program was six years, and the curriculum included 80 percent Chinese medicine and 20 percent Western medicine. (This percentage has been changing in recent years—to 70 percent Chinese and 30 percent Western in most cases—and is different in different schools.) The curriculum stressed the basics of modern anatomy, physiology, pathology, and resuscitation techniques for emergency conditions. The graduated student was approved to practice Chinese medicine (including acupuncture). At the same time, almost the same number of Western-style medical schools appeared or were expanded. These schools also required that students take 10 percent to 20 percent of their required course hours in the area of Chinese medicine.

By the mid-1950s, the government made a full scale commitment to the acceptance and study of Traditional Chinese Medicine, and began requiring modern doctors—even established physicians and medical professors—to study some traditional theory and practice. At the same time, traditional doctors were taught the rudiments of modern Western medicine.

The period from 1950 to 1965 was a progressive time for TCM, despite a two-year setback during Mao's "Great Leap Forward," which caused much turmoil and suspended schooling for almost two years in order for the students to be available to support industry in producing steel. Chinese medical schools continued to graduate students, and the number of health care providers grew.

All these great efforts helped to preserve the traditional medical system in a modern context. Chinese medicine made many contributions to the health care of the Chinese people. In 1955, for example, epidemic encephalitis B occurred in Shijiazhuang, Hebei Province, and in 1966 the same epidemic attacked the Beijing area. These two severe epidemic breakouts were controlled by Chinese medicine based on pure Chinese medical theory. In Shijiazhuang, it was recorded that relatively high curative effects were obtained by using medical herbs, primarily Gypsum Decoction. But in Beijing, when the same prescription was adopted, patients failed to respond. Doctors therefore changed their therapeutic strategies. They began to disperse and relieve the damp and heat, and to dissolve and eliminate the pathogenic dampness with aromatics. The results were striking. Thus it can be explained that although diseases are the same, their epidemic localities and onset seasons can be different, and this affects the way they will respond to treatment. At Shijiazhuang, encephalitis B occurred in summer, while the weather was hot; in Beijing, it occurred in autumn, while the weather was damp due to an unbroken spell of rainfall. Consequently, they could not be treated in the same way. This is an example reflecting the effectiveness of the holistic concept of traditional Chinese medicine.

Acupuncture anesthesia is one of the many inventions that have made Chinese medical practice today unique in the world. It was acupuncture anesthesia that first attracted the attention of foreign doctors to the Chinese medical system. This technique was first tried for painful dressing changes and was also found to be effective in relieving throat pain after tonsillectomies. These observations led doctors to believe that acupuncture might possibly provide anesthesia for surgery.

The year 1958 was a mentally creative time for Chinese people, who were encouraged by the thought of Chairman Mao, who said "All miracle things can be created." People imagined that tons of wheat could be harvested from one acre, and thus neglected their farms, causing thousands of people to die of famine. This type of thinking was encouraged by corrupt local officials. In the case of acupuncture anesthesia, however, those forward-thinking individuals who based their theories in science found this philosophy to be correct and practical. The trial of acupuncture anesthesia for tonsillectomy was successful.

In 1960, however, the use of acupuncture anesthesia was extended to major operations such as lung resection, and many obstacles were encountered. As a result, many doctors began to do basic laboratory research to solve these problems, though their efforts were cut short by the cultural revolution in 1966.

Chinese medicine suffered greatly in the late 1960s, as the educational system was nearly disassembled. Most professors were exiled to rural areas to improve their proletarian thought. Those medical school professors who remained, along with their students, were organized as medical mobile teams to support agriculture by treating workers. The basic theories of Traditional Chinese Medicine were criticized as superstition. Under the cruel pressure of academic reproach and intolerable torture, many physicians committed suicide.

By 1973, some universities and Chinese medical schools (including Western-style medical schools) began enrolling students again, but due to the decline of the educational system, students were admitted to schools based on their political background rather than their intelligence, so the quality of students was poor. The curriculum was reduced to three years, with many important courses eliminated. This condition lasted through 1976. Students who graduated during this time were later called Gong Nong Bing Xue Yuan ("Worker, Peasant and Soldier student"—an uncomplimentary term). However, among these were a few brilliant students, whose contributions cannot be neglected.

"Barefoot Doctors"

Barefoot doctors, who first appeared during the 1960s and 1970s, were physicians who had received limited medical training—typically only a few months to a year—and who lived in rural areas. Their lack of systematic training meant that their treatments were not always effective, and this fact might have contributed to an erroneous reputation for Chinese medicine. But viewed from another angle, due to the barefoot doctors, many people benefitted from Chinese medicine who would not otherwise have received health care. It was convenient, low in cost, and often effective, and it was rooted in the heart of the people.

As time passed, many of the barefoot doctors were gradually replaced by those with more formal training as Chinese physicians. But in many rural areas, barefoot doctors still play a very important role in health care, providing primary health care services for much of the population in China.

In 1977, the entire education system in China was reorganized. Chinese medical schools reinstituted the National Examination, which was held once a year for all high school graduates. Approximately five thousand students were enrolled each year in Chinese medical school to study Chinese medicine. The curriculum differed according to the school, but the basic program was designed for five years of full-time study. Some programs lasted six years. Students coming directly from high school had already been introduced to most scientific subjects, such as physics, chemistry, advanced mathematics, and biology.

In 1983, postgraduate degrees were reinstituted. The full course of Chinese medicine thus consisted of five years of medical school, three years to earn a master's degree, and three years for a doctorate. Students had to pass a written examination and give an oral defense of their research thesis in order to earn their graduate certificate. Although the curriculum varied for degree-seeking postgraduate students, depending on the supervising professor and his specialty, it was recommended that the degree research project should include laboratory work.

The Basic Curriculum of a Traditional Chinese Medical School (1979–1984)

First Year

The Essence and Foundation of Traditional Chinese Medicine (TCM)
Ancient Chinese Literature on TCM
History of TCM
Chinese Materia Medica
The Yellow Emperor's Canon of Internal Medicine
Philosophy

Chinese Phamacology and Formulation Theory
Anatomy

Second Year

Diagnostics of TCM
Treatise on Febrile Disease Caused by Cold
Political Economics
Biochemistry
English
Physiology
Epidemic Febrile Diseases
Physical Education

Third Year

Microbiology & Parasitology
History of Chinese Revolution
Latin
Synopsis of text: "Prescriptions of Golden Chamber"
Pathology

Internship following Professor in hospital for three months

Fourth Year

Science of Acupuncture and Moxibustion
Ophthalmology and Otorhinolaryngology of TCM
Gynecology of TCM
Diagnostics (including all available modern medical diagnostic techniques, such as X ray, ultrasound, and laboratory blood tests)

Pharmacology
Surgery of TCM
Orthopedics and Traumatology of TCM
Internal Medicine of TCM

Fifth Year

Internal Medicine
Surgery
Doctrines of Various TCM Schools
Pediatrics of TCM
Science of Sanitation and Epidemic Prevention

Students were assigned to different hospitals to intern for a total of sixteen months, two months in each of the following departments: cardiovascular, respiratory, blood, digestive disease, surgery, gynecology and obstetrics, neurology, and acupuncture and moxibustion.

When students graduate from medical school, they are licensed to practice Chinese medicine, but it is expected that they will spend one or two years as a resident doctor, supervised by a senior doctor, before beginning an independent practice.

If a licensed Chinese medical practitioner wishes to practice modern (Western) medicine, he can take the required examination to be approved. The same procedure applies for the doctor who graduated from Western medical school who wishes to practice Chinese medicine. Currently, these rules are not strictly adhered to in China.

In the hospitals of China, there are two types of practice. One type consists of mainly modern medicine, similar to the hospitals in the West. The difference lies in the special division established for the practice of Chinese medicine. The patient who is treated under another division of the hospital can be treated with Chinese medicine at the same time. Most of the hospitals in China are run this way. The second type of hospital primarily practices Chinese medicine. They have their own emergency and surgery divisions, and can deal with common diseases—even those that require surgery. The main focus, however, is on traditional Chinese medicine. These hospitals cover many specialties, such as internal medicine, orthopedics, gynecology, pediatrics, and acupuncture and moxibustion.

This health-care system provides the most comprehensive care for the patient. Through experience accumulated over time, China seems to have found the best pattern for health care. It is usually recommended that acute cases, orthopedics cases, emergency cases, and some cases in which surgery is deemed necessary, should be treated with modern medicine. Also, antibiotics, hormone therapy, chemotherapy, and radiotherapy are respected as useful therapies for necessary cases. For most chronic cases, pediatric cases, and gynecological cases, Chinese medicine is the preferred treatment method.

As previously mentioned, there has been much controversy over the position of Traditional Chinese Medicine since Western medicine was first introduced into China. Excluding political prejudice and influence, the real argument about Traditional Chinese Medicine has been whether it has value as a medical science equal to that of Western medicine. This argument may continue as time goes on, but, in my opinion, the balance between Western medicine and Traditional Chinese medicine that has been reached in China at this time reflects the best of both systems. Traditional Chinese medicine has virtues and advantages equaling those of Western medicine. More importantly, because Western medicine does have shortcomings, traditional Chinese medicine can do some things that modern medicine cannot. I believe that both of these medical systems can compensate for the shortcomings of the other.

Modern Applications of Traditional Chinese Medicine

As we have seen throughout this book, Chinese physicians have diligently used the research of their predecessors and their own clinical experience to accurately diagnose and treat disease. Although they have refined their methods over the centuries, the essential procedures for diagnosis and treatment remain the same. In the following chapters, we will show how Traditional Chinese Medicine can be used to treat a number of medical problems for which Western medicine is often only partially successful. Chinese medicine always strives to employ the most useful features of each tradition; thus, Western laboratory tests are often used to confirm the diagnoses of Traditional Chinese Medicine. The next chapter presents the Chinese approach to AIDS, Chronic Fatigue Syndrome, cancer, heart disease, liver disease, arthritis, and diabetes, with some actual case studies from ancient records as well as more recent patients.

Notes

1. In China, no governmental agencies were carried from one dynasty to the next. Each ruler would abolish the governmental structure created by his predecessor and establish his own. The Tang rulers were able to exert such a lasting influence on medical training partly because they were in power for nearly two hundred years—plenty time enough to establish methods and instill attitudes that would influence successive generations of medical practitioners.

2. "Connotation" refers to the practice of curing disease by prayer and incantation—a practice that is mentioned in one of the earliest medical texts, the *Nei Jing*. The fact that doctors accepted this method on an equal basis with more "scientific" methods shows how Chinese medicine treated the whole person by relying on every possible beneficial treatment. Recent Western studies are also beginning to accept the fact that factors other than strict natural science can contribute to cure.

3. The Yuan Dynasty was founded by the Mongols, who invaded China and unified the country under one government for the first time in history.

V
Traditional Chinese Medicine and Western Treatments

13
HIV/AIDS

Chinese Medicine has long recognized the important role of immunology. The history of immunological concepts dates back at least two thousand years. At that time, the immune system was conceived of as a process to resist the entry of evil into the body, contributing not only to health, but also to longevity. From the first vaccination to the evolving theories of pathogens and the many preventive and therapeutic techniques in use by the twentieth century, we can see that Chinese Medicine has successfully reached this goal in its own way.

Chinese Medicine recognizes two primary factors in the study of immunology: 1) the state of the body's resistance and 2) the necessity for expelling pathogens that have succeeded in invading the body.

The relative strength or weakness of the body's resistance determines the likelihood of the pathogen invading the body. Body resistance is a function of the strength of the body's Zheng Qi (vital energy), its Wei Qi (defense energy) and the Qi of all the organs, especially that of the spleen, kidneys, and lungs. The main concern in increasing resistance is how to keep this Qi (energy) at its peak efficiency. Over the years, many theories were tested, including the use of tonic herbal medicine, establishing a proper diet and healthy lifestyle, and so on. The crowning glory of this work was the milestone technique of nasal bovine vaccination for use against smallpox, invented by Chao, in the early portion of the Tang Dynasty.

If pathogens succeed in invading the body, Chinese Medicine prescribes their expulsion through acupuncture, herbal medicine, and even through Qi Gong exercise (see chapter 7). Modern scientific studies, both in pharmacology and physiology, are proving the effectiveness of such treatments for the immune system. To illustrate the logical methodology of TCM and some of the scientific mechanisms underlying why it works, we will discuss the retrovirus HIV and AIDS.

Since AIDS was first discovered to be a contagious and fatal disease, Chinese scientists have done considerable research into solving this problem. Many research groups from China have traveled to areas in which there are numerous AIDS patients to conduct their research. From their many case studies and subsequent publications, we see that treatment with Chinese herbal medicine and acupuncture is extremely encouraging.

Opportunistic infections, which frequently complicate the clinical course of HIV-infected patients, are often the eventual cause of death. To improve and extend the quality of life of the patient, by preventing or eliminating these infections, is the first concern. To prevent the opportunistic infection from taking hold, specific herbal formulas that work toward changing the patient's constitution are prescribed.

Research has shown that many herbal medicines have the ability to boost the body's resistance by protecting the integrity of cellular membranes. Some examples are white peony for liver cells and Chuan Xiong (a Chinese root) for protecting the immune cells. Chuan Xiong is mentioned in the classic herbal texts for its function in treating blood.

Once the HIV virus has entered a cell, a complex sequence of events follows that, if completed, leads to the budding of new virus particles from the infected cell. But when a person acquires an HIV infection, the body initially mounts a vigorous immune defense. During this acute phase of infection, B lymphytes produce antibodies that neutralize the virus, and activated killer T cells multiply and destroy infected cells, much as they would for other diseases. Although it is possible that the immune system may successfully fight off HIV at a very early stage, by the time HIV antibodies are found in the blood, infection is generally permanent.

The clinical picture of acute HIV infections with a mild, flulike illness, accompanied by tiredness and, typically, fever and muscle aches, that usually lasts no more than a few weeks. During this time, large amounts of the virus are present in the bloodstream, and transmission is probably relatively easy. Then the immune response is mounted and begins to eliminate infected cells and the circulating virus. A proportion of infected cells usually remains, however, eluding the host's defenses, and the virus continues to replicate in lower numbers. This stage may last as long as a decade. For most of this period of chronic infection, the patient usually feels quite well. Only after several years does the virus so significantly damage the immune system that opportunistic malignancies and infections appear.

At present, a major concern of those in the medical field is how to prevent those infected with HIV from progressing to full-blown AIDS, as well as how to relieve pain, control symptoms, improve the quality of life of AIDS patients, and treat the common opportunistic infections and cancer associated with AIDS.

Chinese Medicine especially concerned with preventive medicine. It is a famous maxim in TCM that the most respected doctors treat people before they get sick. Besides basic preventive measures such as avoiding the pathogen by avoiding contagious sources, there is the problem that not all people react the same way when exposed to a pathogen. Some people contract symptoms almost immediately, while others may be carriers for years without contracting any symptoms. Therefore, in Chinese medicine, the first concern is to increase resistance. The second is to treat the symptoms and control the opportunistic infections.

It could be said that all care in AIDS is necessarily palliative, since no specific cure has been found. However, some types of Chinese medical intervention can clearly prolong life in HIV- or AIDS-infected patients. Because the disease is newly discovered and those most commonly affected are relatively young, it is natural that medical research and care has been aimed at prolonging life at all costs and in all possible ways.

The clinical manifestation of AIDS are reminiscent of the Yin Yang Yi syndrome, first recorded in *Shang Han Lun Tiao Bian*, ("The Differentiation of Febrile Disease Caused by Cold," published in 1589). Yin Yang Yi syndrome was described as follows: "A febrile disease caused by cold with Yin Yang Yi syndrome will have the following symptoms and signs: a feeling of heaviness in movement, shortness of breath, spasm and an uncomfortable feeling either in the abdomen or even stretching into the genitals, a feeling of heat ascending to the chest, heaviness in the head, a reluctance to lift the head, vertigo, and spasm in the knees and tibia. Shao Kun Powder will be a curative."

The narrative goes on to give instructions for preparing the curing powder. Shao Kun powder is prepared by mixing ashes from burning a piece of cloth taken from a woman's underpants (for a male patient) with water, after taking three doses a day, there will be normal urination and a little swelling over the penis, which is an indication of recovery. (If the patient is a woman, the piece of cloth is taken from a man's underpants.)

"Yin" in this context means woman; "Yang" means man. "Yi" means transferring or infecting. Yin Yang Yi thus means a disease that infects and is transmitted between sexual partners. There is no other relatively modern disease that fits with this disease. It is very clear that Yin Yang Yi is not a very common sexually transmitted disease, and this account, written over four hundred years ago, may refer to one kind of late-stage AIDS syndrome. The strange powder may possess some special value and play an important though indirect role in curing this syndrome.

From another angle, AIDS can be categorized as one type of syndrome of febrile disease caused by pathogenic heat.[1] It fits especially well into the classic three-stage paradigm:

Stage 1. It begins with flulike symptoms, which are classically categorized as pathogenic heat in the defensive (wei) level. The patient's symptoms can be relieved through dispersing the exterior with heat-clearing and detoxifying herbal formulas such as Yin Qiao San (honeysuckle flower and forsythia fruit powder) or Sang Ju Yin (mulberry leaf and chrysanthemum flower decoction).

Stage 2. In the second stage, pathogenic heat blazing upward, the patient may have severe signs, such as PCP (Pneumocystic Carinii Pneumonia) or other types of opportunistic infections, or some neoplasm problem, all of which are explained as toxic accumulation in Chinese Medicine. The therapeutic principle is clearing heat from Qi and blood stage. Bai Hu Tang (white tiger decoction) and Qing Ying Tang will be the best choices.

Stage 3. In the third stage, after suffering many opportunistic infections over time, the patient has no vital energy and is left with a consumptive condition. In one manifestation, the pathogen being so deep inside of the body, the patient may show signs such as severe watery diarrhea without any heat sensation, have a severe headache with no energy to lift his head, and be very thin with atrophied muscles. Or the patient may only feel extremely tired and exhausted. The therapeutic principle will be to disperse the residential pathogen and tonify the energy. The best medical formulas are Zhu Ye Shi Gao Tang (bamboo leaf and gypsum decoction), Mai Men Dong Tang (Ophiopogen Root Decoction) and Bu Yang Huan Wu Tang (Tonifying Yang to Restore Five Organs Decoction).

In the early stage, the HIV carrier with muscle pain will be strongly recommended to be treated with acupuncture at the same time. Overall, however, Chinese herbal medicine is the best solution.

Case 1. Patient XXXX, clinical No. 97. Her first office visit was Jan. 1998. She was one and half years old. Her mother took her to my office. She was a little black girl. She was adopted. She was born HIV positive. Her CD4 count was between 70–90. She was very weak. Her mother was a brilliant and very open-minded lady. I examined the baby. She was physically healthy little girl. The major thing was to improve her CD4 count and prevent the virus from soaring. Chinese medicine has its great advantage in pediatrics. I prescribed my Bing De Ling™ to her. Bing De Ling™ is my personal formula for increasing energy and eliminated toxin. I let her take half ounce each time and two times daily. As soon as she started Bing De Ling™, her CD4 count kept elevating. About two years later, her CD4 count went back to normal. Due to the strong side effect of the anti-virus drug, the patient's mother has never given the baby the drug. She has kept the best record of her daughter's blood test reports. For over seven years, the patient's mom and dad always kept her on the Bing De Ling™, the little girl is now a strong, tall healthy girl. One day the mother said to me, "Dr. Zhao, anytime you want a presentation for this case, I like to go with you to testimony." Prevention is the best way.[2]

Case 2. Patient XXXX, clinical No. 425. A thirty-six-year-old male. May 6, 1999, he was admitted to Sarasota Memorial hospital with severe diarrhea. His treating physician, an infectious disease doctor, referred him to me. There was no medication that could really help his condition. Two years before, he was diagnosed with AIDS. At the moment he had diarrhea twenty-six times per day. The patient was on IV receiving electrolytes and antibiotics. He was very sick. I saw him in the hospital. His temperature was 99°. His height was 5'9". His weight was 116 lbs. His blood pressure was 105/60 mm Hg. He was slim and fragile. His tongue was pale, and his pulse was deep and weak. It had been like this for two weeks. This was definitely a stage three case. Spleen Qi and kidney Qi were very weak as temperature was caused by the Qi deficiency. Diarrhea was led by the weak spleen and kidney not providing energy for digestion and absorbing nutrients. I needed to find a way to increase the spleen and kidney Qi. Chinese medicine formula Bu Zhong Yi Qi Tang (tonify the middle Jiao and increase QI Decoction) was prescribed, which was prepared in liquid form. One batch per day, his relative picked up the herbal medicine for him. After two days of herbal medicine intake, his diarrhea was under control. He was discharged from the hospital. The fourth day, he came to my office by himself to pick up more herbal medicine. His infectious disease doctor was very happy and impressed with the effect of Chinese medicine.

Notes

1. In Chinese medicine, the terms "heat" and "cold" refer not to external feelings of temperature but to specific internal conditions. See chapter 1 for more information.

2. Bing De Ling™ research article has been published in *DNA and Cell Biology,* Volume 19, No. 8, 2000. Pp 515–520.

14
Chronic Fatigue Syndrome

Chronic Fatigue Syndrome (CFS) is a chronic, debilitating illness that affects both men and women. The syndrome is not new, but only in the past eight years has much attention been focused on it by the medical profession.

The current most successful treatment appears to be Polyribonucleotide (Ampligen), an anti-retroviral agent. Unfortunately, it is not currently approved by the FDA, so there is essentially no really effective medicine for this syndrome at this time.

Chinese Medicine examines the entire patient, not just the symptoms. All of these observations are combined and the doctor looks for a pattern. Even if the main complaint is the same, different cases may require different treatments. Following are some examples of different ways in which Chinese Medicine interprets the symptoms of Chronic Fatigue Syndrome:

Mild (Low Grade) Fever has at least three possible causes:

1. Yin Deficiency: the symptom is worse in the afternoon or at night, and the patient has "five heart heat" (a feverish sensation in the palms and soles).
2. Damp invading the body: there is a sensation of congestion and blockage in the chest and stomach, lasting a long time.

3. Middle-jiao Qi deficiency: the symptom is worse after exertion, and is accompanied by abdominal distention and diarrhea.

Recurrent sore throat can be caused by two factors:

1. Heat invading the body: the throat is swollen and red, very painful, and feels soothed when the patient drinks cold liquid. It can be cured without recurrence.
2. Yin deficiency: not very painful but lasting for a long time, coming and going.

Painful Lymph nodes:

1. Blood stasis: the nodes are very hard, painful, and difficult to move.
2. Phlegm: not as hard and easily moved without too much pain, coming and going.

Myalgia (pain in the nerves):

1. Blood statis: very severe fixed pain.
2. Damp invading the body: a heavy and tight feeling over all the body, especially in the lower limbs, lasting for a long time.
3. Qi stagnation: movable pain, worse when emotionally disturbed.

Prolonged fatigue after exercise:

1. Yang deficiency: aversion to cold, temperature sensitive.
2. Qi deficiency: fatigue, no endurance.

Sleep disturbance:

1. Yin Deficiency: difficulty falling asleep, excitable and easily disturbed sleep, restlessness and night sweating.
2. Qi Deficiency: general tiredness, wanting to sleep but having difficulty falling asleep.
3. Inharmonized stomach: stomach distention, much gas.
4. Blood Stasis: pernicious insomnia
5. Liver Yang rising upward: irritability, anger, hypochondriac pain.

From the above analysis, we can see that four pathological conditions seem to explain all the symptoms of Chronic Fatigue Syndrome: Yin and Qi Deficiency, Qi Stagnation, Blood Stagnation, and Damp invading.

Chronic Fatigue Syndrome is a very complex syndrome. In most cases, according to my clinical observations and experience, the above-mentioned four pathologies have been involved. Each case has its own characteristics, and different formulas should be used accordingly. But the above analysis shows that there is a general conceptual formula to build them for chronic fatigue syndrome patients.

The therapeutic principle is aimed at alleviating symptoms and helping patients adjust to the debilitating and chronic nature of the illness. This is accomplished by tonifying the body's Yin and Qi, regulating the Qi's movement, moving blood and promoting blood circulation, and draining/dispelling damp. Any of these methods can be used at same time, and depending on the manifestations, will bring good results if used for a CFS patient.

In choosing which internal organ and channel to treat, I prefer to treat the liver. The liver is the organ responsible for storing blood, so blood deficiency and blood stasis are related to the liver; it is also responsible for regulating whole body's energy, as it is the main organ to cause the Qi stagnation.

Treatments for CFS

Herbal medicines allow for a very flexible treatment plan. You can design a formula for each patient according to the peculiarities of each case. There are herbs to tonify Yin and Qi, to regulate the Qi and move blood, and to drain/dispel damp. The herbs are organized into a formula according to special rules and ratios.

Use of special points and types of manipulations with acupuncture can achieve many of the same functions as provided by herbal medicine.

The ancient method of moxibustion is a very powerful way to increase energy, but it creates a smoky environment in the clinic. A Biofrequency Spectrum Therapeutic Device can now be used to replace moxibustion treatment.

Prognosis

Any kind of therapy for CFS will take time—at least two or three months. During the treatment, there will be four to five instances when the symptoms return strongly. It is important to counsel the patient not to become discouraged during bad times and not to become overly optimistic during the good times. However, this is definitely a disease that can be cured.

Ancient Records Relating to CFS

Ancient Chinese medical texts contain many descriptions of syndromes that are more than 98 percent similar to CFS, and include treatment protocols as well. In different texts, this syndrome is variously referred to as Yin Yang Du (both Yin and Yang are toxicated) syndrome, Hu Huo (toxicated by fox) syndrome, Xu Sun (deficiency and damage) syndrome, or Xu Lao (deficiency tiredness) syndrome.

Jin Gui Yao Lie ("Synopsis of Prescriptions of the Golden Chamber"), one of the great classics of TCM, was written in the second or third century by the great doctor Zhang Zhong Jing. It is the earliest extended treatise on miscellaneous diseases. In this book he described three different syndromes:

1. Bai He (Bulbous Lilii) Syndrome: Symptoms and signs of this syndrome may include: the patient wants to eat, but is reluctant to swallow food and is unwilling to speak. Or he prefers to lie in bed, yet cannot lie quietly due to restlessness. He may want to walk about, but soon becomes tired. Now and then he may enjoy eating certain delicacies, but at other times he cannot even tolerate the smell of food. He may feel either cold and hot, but without discernible fever or chill. He may also have a bitter taste in his mouth and pass reddish urine. No medicine appears able to cure the syndrome. After taking medicine, acute vomiting and diarrhea may occur. The disease "haunts" the patient, and though his appearance is normal, he is actually suffering. His pulse is somewhat speedy. The Decoction Bulbous Lilli and Radix Rehmanniae (Bai He Di Huang Tang) will be effective in curing the case.

2. Hu Huo Syndrome: Symptoms and signs are similar to those of febrile diseases caused by cold. The patient is reluctant to speak and tends to sleep. But he cannot shut his eyes when he feels restless. When ulceration appears in the throat, this is Huo syndrome: When ulceration appears on external genitals, it is a Hu syndrome. Reluctance to eat, aversion to food odors, facial complexion occasionally red, sometimes black or pale. Decoction Radix Glycyrrhizae Xienin can be adopted.

3. Xu Lao (Consumptive) Syndrome. Patient will feel tired and begin to sweat after working for a short time. When he lies in bed, he will toss and turn frequently. If he is exposed to a breeze at this time, he will suffer from arthralgia due to stagnation of blood. The pulse will be feeble and hesitant and slender-tense at Cun Kou. Acupuncture therapy can be adopted to stimulate the Yang Vital Energy. Decoction Five herbs with Radix Astragali and Ramulus Cinnamomi will provide a cure.

Consumptive diseases in male and female patients have the following symptoms and signs: Owning to accumulation of chronic pathogenic cold and stagnation of Vital Energy, the patient suffers from heaviness in the extremities, weakness and aching in bones and muscles, difficulty breathing, wheezing and fatigue when moving around, a sense of fullness in the chest and a feeling of adverse ascending air (acid reflux and hiccups) stiffness and pain in the back and the waist, palpitations, parched lips and throat, dark facial and skin complexion, poor appetite, distention in the chest, coastal regions and abdomen, difficulty in lifting the head, and preference for lying down. After the disease lasts a hundred days or more, the patient becomes thin and weak. When the Vital Energy of the Five Viscera is exhausted, recovery is difficult. Pulses on the inch, bar and cubit[1] of both wrists are deficient and weak, and deficiency and cold prevail. Patient feels a lack of vitality, with constant abdominal contraction and numerous other symptoms of a deficient nature. Decoction Radix Astragali Jian Zhong will be adopted for this syndrome.

It is clear from these extensive descriptions that Dr. Zhang recognized, even at this early point in history, that this syndrome can have several different clinical appearances. Following the tenants of TCM, he designed many formulas for different types of patients, leaving a valuable legacy for future generations of physicians.

Another case that seems most similar to Chronic Fatigue Syndrome is found in *Ming Yi Lei An* ("The Classified Cases of Famous Doctors"), which was published during the Ming Dynasty (1540 A.D.). A case treated by Dr. Luo was recorded in detail as follows.

Dr. Luo treated a 23-year-old patient, Zhou Qing Zi, who was a district officer in the government. During the spring season, he suffered from fever, loss of weight, lassitude of the four limbs, sleeping continuously, night sweating, loose bowels and diarrhea with rattling sound in the abdomen, no appetite, no ability to taste food, and too tired to speak. These symptoms came and went for over a half year. Dr. Luo found the patient had a floating pulse and diagnosed, "There was cold accumulated in the internal organ with the heat in the blood."

His first treatment was to increase the deficiency with moxibustion on various acupoints to induce the clear Qi upward, nourish the original Qi, and promote muscle regeneration. Second, he used Jing Mi (Oryza rice), Fu Ling (Poria), Tian Dong (asparagus root) and other remedies to "clear heat" and "warm the cold." The disease was under control in three months, and after two years, the patient had become very strong and gained weight. According to the patient's disease history, symptoms, and signs of Mr. Zhou, he appears to have suffered from Chronic Fatigue Syndrome.

Notes

1. See chapter (4) for discussion of the divisions of the pulse.

15
Cancer

Cancer and malignant tumors were recognized in Chinese medicine at a very early time, being recorded as far back as the Han Dynasty (200 A.D.). In Chinese medicine, cancer and malignant tumor were generally named Ji Ju and Zheng Jia. The first cancers recognized seem to have been the malignant lymphoma and abdominal malignant tumors. They were called Luo Li (lymphoma), Chang Tan (Intestine Tumor), Shi Jia (Tumor hardness like stone, which is liver cancer), or Fan Hua Chuang (tumor looks like a flower blossoming, referring to skin and breast cancer).

In the Song Dynasty (1100), *Wei Ji Bao Shu* clearly used the Chinese character "Ai," which directly translates to "cancer," specifically referring to the malignant tumor as opposed to the benign tumor or abscess/carbuncle. The author correctly stated that breast cancer mostly happens in women over forty, taking about three years to become terminal. In 1264, Dr. Yang Ren Zai published his book *Ren Zai Zhi Zhi Fang*, in which the clinical manifestations and signs of breast cancer were described more clearly and therapeutic formulas were recommended. The first herbal formula principles for treating cancer can be traced back to *Shen Nong Ben Cao Jing*, the first pharmacopoeia (see chapter 5), which stated that all the salty property medicines could be used to soften the tumor (mass).

Tumors and cancer in general were explained in the early pathology of Chinese medicine as something accumulated or obstructed in the local tissue; this was identified with phelgm and stasis blood. Phlegm and blood stasis syndromes in Chinese medicine are among the more difficult syndromes to be treated—even under normal circumstances. These two syndromes can be categorized in three degrees, the third and most severe of which is the malignant tumor/cancer. This is why, in the earliest medical documents, the Ji Ju and Zheng Jia were considered untreatable diseases. By the Song Dynasty (960–1279), especially with the publication of *Sheng Ji Zong Lu* ("Charity General Collection"), the largest collection of formulas for internal medicine, it is clear from the number of formulas listed for malignant tumors that the pathological theory of the disease was becoming more complex.

Pathological Theory

Chinese medicine defined the general pathology of cancer as a combination of the results of phlegm accumulation, blood stasis, and Qi (vital energy) body fluid deficiency.

1. The formation of phlegm: Phlegm is a pathogen, which blocks the movement of energy and blood to cause the tumor. But phlegm itself is a pathological product; it can be caused by spleen energy deficiency or kidney energy deficiency. Because of the underlying deficiency, water retention occurs, and if the body stays in this condition long enough, the retained water is concentrated by heat (from liver or another way) into phlegm. Phlegm can be transported and stored in the lung to be expectorated out, or it can remain anywhere of the body. Wherever the phlegm accumulates, the tumor can form.

2. Blood Stasis: Blood circulation is dominated by the heart, but the spleen and liver also play an important function in this, according to Chinese medical theory. Spleen helps maintain the blood inside the vessels and the liver can regulate the blood.

3. Deficiency syndrome: After a long while, the phlegm and blood stasis obstruct the energy, and blood can not move smoothly. All of the organs and tissues depend on the blood and energy for nourishment. This places the entire body in a deficiency condition, which explains the consumptive nature of the end stage of cancer.

Most of the anti-tumor medicinal formulas targeted these three pathological steps, with more or less specific anti-tumor/cancer medicines added.

Differentiation and Therapeutic Modalities

Cancerous tumors were usually classified into three stages to treat: initial stage, second stage (also named acute stage), and end stage.

In the initial stage, the pathogen is not as deadly. The body's Zheng Qi (vital energy) is still strong, as the immune function begins to engage the pathogens. At this point it is quite possible to expel the pathogen and save the patient's life, either through surgery, herbal medicine, or both. To get rid of the pathogen, purgative, diaphoretic, and clear heat and detoxify medicines will be the first group to be used.

In the second stage, clinical manifestations are more severe, with the patient always feeling ill. The pathogen is getting stronger, and the body's resistance (immune function) is getting weaker. The therapeutic principle is adjusted to getting rid of pathogens and at the same time increasing the body's energy (resistance). Besides the above medicines for the first stage, more tonifying Qi and Yin medicine will be used in the prescription. The general formula is: Shi Quan Da Bu Tang (big tonic with ten ingredients).

In the end stage, most patients already have been through chemotherapy or radiation therapy. The patient is exhausted, having no energy, tired, low function of internal organs, no appetite, insomnia, depression, anxiety, hair loss, nausea, weight loss, and many consumptive manifestations. To increase the Qi and Yin is the major concern and principle. This can counteract the side effects and improve the patient's quality of life.

Modern Pharmacological Research on Improving the Function of the Immune System

Through countless generations of clinical experimentation, the effectiveness of herbal medicine has been proven. But given the outlook of modern science, which demands an understanding of the chemical mechanisms involved in their effectiveness, the Chinese government has, for the past ten years, been investing a great deal of time and money in research to answer these questions and perhaps extract the purified substances.

Some of the recently published scientific reports are summarized in the following items.

1. Some herbal medicines, such as Ban Bian Lian, Ban Zhi Lian, or Bai Hua She She Cao, were shown to directly kill the tumor cell in vitro and in vivo. Also it is reported most of the "clear heat" herbs can limit the tumor's metastasis.

2. Some herbal medicines can activate the production of cytokines by T cells such as Huang Qi, Nu Zheng Zi, Du Zhong, and Yin Yang Huo.

3. Herbs such as Huang Qi, Shan Yu Rou, and Gu Sui Bu promote the production of antibodies against tumor cells and promote the production of immune complex formation.

4. Herbs such as Tian San Qi, Ci Wu Jia, and Bei Sha Shen can limit the production of antibodies that cannot recognize normal tissue. This is why herbal medicine has been shown to help auto-immune disease patients.

5. Herbs such as Dang Gui, Chuan Xiong, Lu Jiao Jiao, and E Jiao can promote the production of red and white blood cells, the blood platelet count, and also improve the hemoglobin value.

6. Herbs such as Ye Ju Hua and Hu Lu Ba can greatly improve kidney function.

Case Studies: Malignant Anemia; Leukemia; Brain Cancer with Chemotherapy

The first two cases described below involved patients whom I encountered while practicing in China. The third is a fairly recent case involving a patient seen at my clinic in the United States.

Case 1. A 32-year-old man suffered from headaches for three months. Results of a bone biopsy indicated a diagnosis of malignant anemia and AIH (red blood cell resolved) syndrome, but the pathogensis was not clear. Many treatments were done without results. The patient's clinical manifestations were headache, dizziness, severe fatigue, dark urine, shortness of breath, palpitations, whole body aching, and hemoglobin value of 5. He was undergoing a blood transfusion every two weeks.

After the physical examination, I diagnosed that his problem was caused by kidney energy deficiency. I gave him a formula consisting of ten herbs and instructed him to drink the liquid for ten days. Ten days later, he felt much stronger and felt no side effects. He was instructed to continue the herbal medicine for another two months. During that time, he did not receive any blood transfusion, and his hemoglobin level reached 13. That was five years ago. I recently received a letter from a friend in China mentioning this patient. His health condition is very good, and he continues to drink the herbal preparation for ten days every two months. He takes that formula as his life.

Case 2. A three-year-old boy had suffered from high fever (39–40 C) for a month. A blood test indicated that his white blood cell count was 34,000. Biopsy pathology confirmed this result. He was diagnosed with acute granular leukemia. His parents brought him to consult with my professor and me. "This fever is caused by the heat accumulated inside," my professor decided after checking the boy's pulse and tongue. He focused on the boy's fever, because that was his main symptom. So we prescribed a formula consisting of seven herbs, with low dosage due to his age. Three days later, we checked him again. His temperature was down to 37–38 C. Continuing this formula for eleven months, the boy's fever declined to a normal range. The white blood cell count went down to 5,000. A Chinese newspaper celebrated this successful case with a prominent article headlined "Herbal Medicine Can Cure Leukemia."

Case 3. The patient is a 34-year-old man specializing in computer science. He came from Shang Hai to finish his master's degree at Minnesota University. In September 1992, he found his right limbs numb and had no energy. First he visited a neurologist, who found nothing wrong and told him to do more exercise to promote the blood circulation. But a week later his symptoms got worse. A CT scan and MRI indicated inoperable brain cancer, and his doctor told him he had one month to live. He was started on a heavy course of chemotherapy. After two weeks, his white blood cell count was down to 300—sometimes as low as 100. Stopping the chemotherapy would mean death.

When the patient presented himself at my clinic, I observed that he was very tall (six feet), had a pale complexion, was weak, spoke with a low voice, and had a fresh red tongue and a thin and thready pulse. This syndrome is a Yin Deficiency with Damp Heat inside the patient's body. A formula to increase his Yin, clear the Heat, and drain the Damp was prescribed for him. He was to drink this herbal medicine and continue his chemotherapy. He bought a two-month supply of herbs from Chinatown in New York City and kept in contact by phone every week. Soon the patient felt progressive improvement. After three weeks, the blood test reported a white blood cell count of 3,300. The patient continued to improve and by July 1993 had moved back to China, apparently healthy.

Chemotherapy and radiation therapy can cause the body to lose a lot of body fluid that is classified as Yin. The therapies themselves are toxic, which is a manifestation of heat. Therefore, correcting the side effects of chemotherapy and radiation therapy focuses on increasing the Yin of the kidney and clearing heat.

The therapeutic principles for cancer patients undergoing chemotherapy and radiotherapy is thus to:

Tonify Kidney Yin & Blood with formulas such as Yin Yang Huo, Gou Qi Zi, Nu Zheng Zi, Han Lian Cao, Shan Zhu Yu, Dang Gui, and Dan Shen.

Clear Heat with formulas such as Huang Qin, Huang Lian, Huang Bai, Zhi Mu, Ban Zhi Lian, Ban Bian Lian, and Bai Hua She She Cao.

Sometimes it is best to add some herbs to increase energy (Huang Qi, Ren Shen) or drain damp (Fu Ling, Bai Zhu, Ze Xie), as required.

The treatment protocol calls for oral administration of the herbal medicine in liquid, powder, or capsule. Usually, in the beginning, the liquid form is used, because it is more powerful. These herbs have no side effects. They don't upset the patient's stomach and, in fact, actually help prevent the damage that chemotherapy causes to the stomach.

16

Diabetes Mellitus

Diabetes mellitus is named Xiao Ke (wasting and thirsting syndrome) in Chinese medicine. This name first appears in the great Dr. Zhang's *Jin Gui Yao Lue* ("Synopsis of Prescriptions of the Golden Chamber—see page 12). It was described thus: "Patient has frequent urination. When he drinks———of water, he passes as much as———of urine. Pills of Eight Ingredients of Kidney Vital Energy can be adopted.

Considering the different patterns of diabetes, the pathologies vary: If the case caused accumulation of pathogenic heat in the middle portion (the stomach), it is called Middle Xiao Ke (Zhong Xiao). If the failure of the deficient Kidney Yang Vital Energy to evaporate the body fluid has resulted in a failure to bring the fluid upward, which in turn causes an inability to control urination due to poor circulation of the vital energy, it is called Lower Xiao Ke (Xia Xiao). If the pathogenic heat stays in the lung and exhausts the body fluid to cause great thirst. It is called upper Xiao Ke (Shang Xiao). Later, in the Tang Dynasty (c. 630 A.D.), it was recognized that a diabetic patient's urine is sweet, contains sugar, and therefore is liked by ants.

The pathology and therapy for diabetes has became very well understood in the present. It is interesting to note that, despite all the refinements of later years, the clinical patterns of diabetes follow the original pattern laid out by Zhang Zhong Jing, in which diabetes was classified into three patterns: Upper

Xiao Ke—Disorder of the lung; Middle Xiao Ke—Disorder of the stomach; Lower Xiao Ke—Disorder of the kidney.

In Chinese medicine, sugar or protein loss and frequent urination were considered the misfunctioning of the water gate, which is caused by deficiency of the kidney's vital energy. Thirst indicates body fluid deficiency, but this can be caused by either of two factors: one is the pathogenic heat burning the body fluid in stomach/lung, and the other is the spleen and stomach not performing their function of absorbing and transporting fluid. Based on these facts, it is easy to understand the therapeutic principle for diabetes in Chinese medicine: to clear the pathogenic heat from the body, increase the body fluid, and increase the vital energy of the kidney and spleen. Herbal medicine, acupuncture, and moxibustion modalities can bring the body back into balance.

To practice Chinese medicine in U.S., you have to modify the therapy based on the whole environment. Most diabetes patients are already getting medical care, with variety medications, such as Glucotrol or Glucophage, or insulin. In this situation, we wonder if it is necessary to seek Chinese medicine. The answer is yes. It is still very necessary to get help from Chinese medicine. First, for diabetes I, insulin dependent case, many patients may develop insulin resistance. So to prevent this nasty condition, the best way is to not abuse the insulin. To use more natural medicine help to increase the liver function, which can help the glucose and glucogen transformation procedure. Many herbal medicines which can keep the liver QI flow smoothly, can lower the blood sugar level. Acupuncture to stimulate Liv. 14, Liv 13, Ren. 12 can also help the whole situation. In many cases, a patient's insulin dosage was reduced significantly.

Secondly, there are the complications from diabetes, such as retinopathy, neuropathy, nephropathy, cardiovascular disorder and hypertension. Acupuncture and herbal medicine may be the best modalities for controlling these complications in clinical practice. But as a practitioner, your treatment has to be based on the individual patient's clinical manifestation.

17
Liver Diseases (Hepatitis B, Hepatitis C, Alcohol/Drug Induced Liver Damage and Liver Cirrhosis)

There is evidence that Chinese doctors recognized hepatitis as early as the third century. The condition was first described as Huang Dan (jaundice), or hypochondriac pain. The symptoms and clinical manifestations were identified in *Shang Han Lun* written during the Han Dynasty (c. 220 A.D.) and later in *Zhu Bing Yuan Hou Lun* (Sui Dynasty, c. 560 A.D.). Jaundice and hypochondriac pain were eventually directly related to the function of the liver. Damp and heat were thought to be the major pathogens. The theory was that damp and heat invade the liver, blocking the movement of liver Qi and gall bile; the accumulated bile then leaks into the bloodstream, causing the jaundice and hypochondriac pain.

If the jaundice and hypochondriac pain cannot be cured, the disease progresses from liver Qi stagnation to blood stasis and then to Yin deficiency, when it manifests as liver fibrosis and liver cirrhosis. In Chinese medicine, liver cirrhosis was variously called Gan Shui (liver edema), Zheng Jia (mass), Ji Ju (lump), and Fei Qi (fatty liver).

The symptoms of liver cirrhosis were described as Gan Shui (liver edema) in *Jin Gui Yao Lue* ("Symposium of the Golden Chamber," 220 A.D.). The ascite (water build-up in the pelvic cavity) of abdominal cavity was first related to liver function disorder. Surely, at that time, the author was not aware that this was caused by low albumin in bloodstream, but his deductions based on simple observation were brilliant.

The physician best known for treating liver disease is Zhang Lu (Qing Dynasty), who wrote *Zhang Shi Yi Tong* ("Doctor Zhang's Medical Theories," published 1695). His book describes many excellent formulas for treating liver disease. The most popular formula for this condition is the Xiao Chai Hu Tang (minor bupleum root decoction), and the best formula for treating jaundice is Yin Chen Hao Tang (sweet evergreen worm decoction), both of which were invented by Dr. Zhang Zhong Jing, who lived in the 3rd century A.D.

In my own research and clinical experience, I have categorized liver disease into four stages, each with a particular diagnosis and treatment:

1. Liver Qi (energy) stagnation. This type covers the early and chronic prolonged stages of Hepatitis B and Hepatitis C. The patient suffers low energy and fatigue, and hypochondriac pain; he or she has no appetite, sighs frequently, has a wiry pulse, and the tongue has a white and sticky coating. Blood tests such as SGPT, SGOT, GGP, Total Bilirubin, LDH, and so on may show a high value for the liver enzyme, while other markers remain in normal range. Virus immunological markers, such as HBsAg, HbeAg, and HbcAg, should be positive.

In this condition, only the Qi movement is affected, so treatment aims to move and regulate the liver energy while at the same time clearing liver heat. The medicinal formulas used are Xiao Chai Hu Tang (decoction of minor bupleurum combination) and Hao Qin Qing Dan Tang (febrifugal decoction of sweet wormwood and scutellaria combination).

2. Damp and heat in liver. This pattern includes chronic active hepatitis (B & C). In this condition, the patient may have jaundice, fever, hypochondriac pain, severe nausea, vomiting,

an aversion to greasy food, extreme tiredness or achiness all over the body. Blood tests show an elevated serum enzyme value and the positive hepatitis virus B/C antigens and antibodies. The pulse is wiry and rapid. The tongue is red and has a thick, yellow coating.

The therapeutic principle is to clear the damp-heat from liver and gall bladder and to stop the disease progression. The formula used is Yin Chen Hao Tang (decoction herba artemisiae scopariae). This is one of the formulas originated by Dr. Zhang Zhong Jin in the 3rd century. Dr. Zhang's book states: "The patient has fever and chills and is reluctant to eat. If he eats, he will experience vertigo and uneasiness in his chest. This condition will last for a period of time after which his skin will turn yellow. This is jaundice due to improper diet. Yin Chen Hao Tang can be adopted." No better formula for jaundice has been discovered since Dr. Zhang's day.

3. Spleen Qi deficiency: Due to the lack of an effective treatment for chronic Hepatitis B/C, most cases last for quite a long time. At this third, prolonged stage, the pathology changes from damp-heat accumulated in liver to spleen Qi deficiency. The clinical manifestations are a pale complexion, fatigue, no appetite, loose bowel movements or watery diarrhea, a big, pale tongue showing toothmarks, and a soft and weak pulse.

The therapeutic principle is to increase the spleen energy while at the same time clearing the damp-heat from the liver channel, which was thought to be the residual pathogen. The formula used is Chai Hu Gui Zhi Gan Jiang Tang (decoction radix bupleuri, ramulus cinnamoni and rhizoma zingiberis). This formula also originated from Dr. Zhang's work. It is a very practical formula that is used in current clinical practice.

4. Complex syndrome of Yin deficiency, damp and heat accumulation and blood stasis: This is the end stage of liver

disease, which can be liver fibrosis or cirrhosis, or even hepatoma. By this time, the patient has been discharged from hospital as a hopeless case. The patient's liver function is on the edge of failure. No real treatment for this stage is available in modern medicine The only treatment that may help is to correct the nutrients and regulate the electrolytes. The patient often suffers ascite, has jaundice (dark and yellow color), has lost a great deal of weight, and is extremely tired. A blood test will show that the ratio of albumin to globumin is reversed. The serum enzyme is not very high, except perhaps GGTP. The patient's tongue may be purple, or have many black spots without a coating, or it may appear fresh and red without a coating (called "mirror tongue," a sign of Yin deficiency). Most patients exhibit enlarged or radiating blood vessels, which look like stars on the surface of the chest or upper body.

In this stage, the basic pathology of liver cirrhosis is very complicated, including the Qi stagnation, damp and heat invading, blood stasis, and blood and Yin deficiency; some cases also show the Yang Qi deficiency. Liver cirrhosis is difficult to treat. The therapeutic principle is to regulate liver Qi, move blood, clear damp and heat, and tonify the body's Yin/Yang, all at the same time. The formula used is Qing Hao Bie Jia Tang (decoction of sweet wormwood and tortoise shell). If the patient's ascites is the major complaint, Fu Ling (Poria), Zhu Ling (Umbellate pore-fungus), Ze Xie (Alismatis rhizoma), Bin Lang (Betel nut), and Dong Gua Pi (Benincasa peel) are added to the above formula. Often, I combine this formula with another patent Chinese herbal medicine named Bie Ja Jian Wan (tortoise shell pill) or Pain Zi Huang.

Using these medicines, the effective cure rate can be as high as 75 percent. The treatment course should run about six months.

Precautions: Liver disease patients in any stage, no drinking of alcohol, overwork, or emotional disturbance can be allowed. Even one of these factors can block the therapy and worsen the condition.

18
Heart Disease

Angina and atherosclerosis were recognized in China as early as the 7th century A.D. by Dr. Sun Xi Miao. In *Jin Gui Yao Lie*, it was called Xiong Bi, which means the chest blocked by phlegm with chest Yang deficiency. Phlegm is one of the secondary pathogens, which can remain in the channel/meridians of the heart.

From the Han to the Tang dynasties in clinical practice, many greatly effective medicinal formulas were discovered. According to the clinical experience of Professor Du Zhou Liu, Ginshen and cinnamon twig are the best herbal medicines for heart disease. Ginshen is good for the weak heart function and can be used in treating congestive heart failure, for example, to increase the output value of the heart. Cinnamon Twig is the best herbal medicine for an irregular heartbeat of any type. Both of these medicines were created by Dr. Zhang Zhong Jing in the 3rd century A.D., and are mentioned in his *Shang Han Lun* ("Treatise on Febrile Disease Caused by Cold"). Another well-known formula for this condition is Zhi Gan Cao Tang (decoction of baked licorice root).

In the 6th century, the great doctor Sun Xi Miao improved on Dr. Zhang's theory and created more practical formulas in his *Qian Jin Yao Fang* ("A Thousand Golden Formulas"), such as Qian Hu Tang Fang (decoction of peucedanum root) designed specifically for left chest tightness and pain. More formulas were developed over the next several centuries.

To simplify this discussion, I will classify the all the heart diseases that we encounter in normal clinical practice into two categories:

1. Heart Qi Deficiency: The patient has a very pale complexion, tiredness, heart palpitation, occasional dizziness, edema in the ankles, a very pale/watery tongue, and a weak or irregular pulse. This condition also includes those patients who have already had the heart bypass surgery.

The therapeutic principle is to increase the heart energy. The main formula used is Zhi Gan Cao Tang (decoction of baked licorice combination).

2. Heart Yang Obstruction Syndrome: The patient complains of chest (left side) stiffness and pain. In some cases, this pain can radiate to the left shoulder and upper back. Extremities are cold. Many of these patients are overweight. The tongue is pale and slippery, and the pulse is irregular or tight. This syndrome caused by phlegm accumulating in the chest and blocking the chest Yang. Coronary artery problems are within this type.

The therapeutic principle is to unblock the chest Yang and transform the phlegm. The formula used is Zhi Shi Xie Bai Gui Zhi Tang (decoction of immature bitter orange, macrostem onion, and cinnamon twig combination).

Depending on individual constitutions, this formula can be modified. If patient's tongue has purple spots or is black, medicines to move the blood (increase the blood circulation) should be added in, such as Dan Shen (Sebaria Ginshen root), Chi Shao Yao (Red Peaonia), and Dan Pi (Moutan bark).

A Note on the Secondary Pathogens Related to Heart Disease

Blood Stasis: Many pathogens can cause poor circulation and blood stasis. Stagnated blood causes the energy movement to be blocked. Masses, lumps, and tumors can be directly blamed on blood stasis. In this case, stagnated blood is both the cause and manifestation of the problem. The major therapeutic principle in treatment is always to move the blood and disperse the stagnated blood.

Phlegm: On the surface, this appears like blood stasis. As a secondary pathogen, phlegm is caused primarily by water retention, which may result from spleen or kidney Qi deficiency. Furthermore, phlegm can travel or stay in one place in the body to block energy movement, leading to tumors or cancer. Treatment concerns are how to transform or get rid of phlegm.

19
Arthritis

Osteoarthritis, rheumatism, and rheumatoid arthritis are included in this category of disease. In Chinese medicine, all these diseases are categorized in Bi syndrome (obstruction syndrome). Bi syndrome was first mentioned in the *Nei Jing*. This treatise classified the Bi syndrome into three different patterns: Xing (moving) Bi, Tong (painful) Bi, and Zhuo (prolonged) Bi. During the Han Dynasty, Dr. Zhang Zhong Jing's book included a special discussion of problems of the joints, stating the clinical manifestations, symptoms, and therapeutic medicinal formulas for arthritis. His formulas are still used in clinical practice with a very good result. The pathology and treatment of arthritis have improved with every succeeding generation.

The major pathogen causing arthritis has always been thought to be damp; therefore, expelling damp is always the main therapeutic principle. Medicinal formulas always include a few ingredients designed to expel and transform the dampness. Damp as a pathogen can invade the body through a humid environment. Additionally, looking at the body's microenvironment, conditions such as overwork can cause spleen Qi deficiency, which governs the function of transportation of water. With this condition, waste water accumulates inside and blocks the channel/meridians, triggering the arthritis. Dr. Zhang Zhong Jing believed that the basic causes of arthritis are the deficiency of liver, kidney, blood, and Qi. In clinical practice, according to the varied pathogens, affected joints, and the patient's constitution, arthritis has been described and treated according to the following patterns:

1. Damp and Heat Bi Syndrome: This type includes the rheumatoid and rheumatic arthritis. The clinical manifestations are swollen and red joints, deformed joints, and fever. The condition is acute and progressive, the patient's pulse is rapid and rolling, and the tongue is red with a sticky coating.

The therapeutic principle is to clear heat and expel the turbid dampness. The medicinal formula prescribed is Jue Bi Tang.

2. Blood cold and Kidney Qi deficiency Bi Syndrome: This type includes the chronic arthritis and osteoarthritis. The patient's symptoms come and go unpredictably, the extremities are very cold, joints are not swollen, there is some old deformity and no fever, the patient likes to be warmed. The pulse is slow and the tongue pale. All the symptoms worsen in a cold and damp environment.

The therapeutic principle is to warm the blood, increase kidney energy, and transform damp. The medicinal formula used is Du Huo Ji Sheng Wan (a patent medicine).

Besides the oral medicine, which treats the cause of the disease, arthritis patients benefit from combinations of acupuncture, moxibustion therapy, external herbal oil massage, medicinal bath, steaming the affected joints with herbal medicine, herbal patches, and other treatments to help reduce the loss of joint flexibility. The pain and suffering of arthritis can be quickly controlled using a variety of treatments.

20

An Ideal Medical Model: Integrating Chinese Medical Philosophies & Ethics into the Current Healthcare System

Abstract

This paper discusses ways in which advantages offered by Chinese medical philosophies and ethics can rectify shortcomings in the prevailing biomedical model. Supporting his argument with case studies drawn from his experience practicing medicine in the United States, the author proposes a new holistic medical model that will involve multi-dimensional thinking and varied therapeutic modalities, and will allow patients to receive maximum benefit from modern medical techniques.

Several fundamental concepts from Chinese medicine and ethics are advanced as part of the new model. Recognizing that the human body is inseparable from nature and thus affected by factors such as climate and weather, season, and time will allow considerations of geography and chronologically in assessing treatments. Accepting the body as a single, inseparable unit when designing therapies will help to reduce trauma and destruction ensuing from single-focus therapies, and restore balance to the interrelationships of the body's organ systems. And finally, a renewed consideration of medical ethics will greatly benefit the relationship between doctor and patient.

❖   ❖   ❖

I have practiced Chinese medicine in the United States for the past five years. During that time, I have encountered a great number of cases that have caused me to very seriously weigh both the advantages and the shortcomings of the current American healthcare system against the practice of Traditional Chinese Medicine.[1] Chinese medicine and Western (modern) Medicine represent two totally different healthcare systems, the first being based on synthesis, the latter on deduction.

The best comparison is Quantum physics versa Newtonian physics. Also Chinese Medicine is the only existing all-encompassing, total health-care system that exists outside the Western Hemisphere.

Modern biomedicine has recently made great advances, especially in surgical techniques and emergency management. But its conceptual framework limits its best performance. The advantage of Chinese medicine lies in dealing with pernicious and chronic diseases by means of regulating the body's natural healing process. Because of its theory and philosophy, this ancient practice continues to shine in the modern era, despite the fact that its therapeutic modalities appear to be old and unsophisticated. Of course, one shortcoming of Chinese medicine lies in dealing with emergency cases and surgical techniques. Currently, using Chinese medicine as a complementary medicine is, at the very least, an improvement over the uni-dimensionality of the biomedical model. But, as I have found in my clinical practice—the idea of Chinese medicine as *complementary* medicine is not enough.

We should establish a *comprehensive* medical model, in which the current modern biomedical model and the essence of Chinese medical philosophy and ethics are merged into a new system. This will equip advanced scientific medical techniques with an organically brilliant humanistic mind. Modern medicine can then achieve its best, most efficient performance. As Dr. Capra (1985) said in his foreword to *Space, Time & Medicine,* the time to do this project is right now:

> In spite of the great advances of modern medical science we are now witnessing a profound crisis in healthcare in Europe and North America . . . perceive the shortcomings of the current healthcare system as being rooted in the conceptual framework that supports medical theory and practice, and have come to believe that the crisis will persist unless this framework is modified . . ., what we need is a new vision of reality, a fundamental change.

As Dr. Capra correctly observed: this is already a real social crisis. Dissatisfied with the current health-care system, many people have searched for alternative medical treatment. This is an objective fact.

Nature and Humankind Correspond to Each Other

—Living beings cannot exist separate from nature.

Chinese view the individual as a microcosm: a reflection of the surrounding universal macrocosm. The principles of universal energy flow are embodied in the inner workings of human beings. From the Chinese philosophical viewpoint, a healthy life is one in which the forces of Yin and Yang are evenly balanced. An imbalance of these polar energies causes a shift in the organism's equilibrium, which ultimately coalesces into patterns of disharmony and illness in the physical body.

Climate
Living in a material world, human bodies are affected in many ways by weather and climate. I have encountered many

cases in which individuals found that their bodies began to deteriorate as soon as they moved to Florida. Typical symptoms were ankle edema, chest stiffness, and skin lesion—all appearing without apparent cause. The individuals who came to my office had already undergone numerous examinations and been told that modern medicine could do nothing for them. This put them under pressure to look for relief in so-called "alternative medicine."

These patients wanted to live in Florida, even though they recognized that their symptoms were related to Florida's humidity and hot weather. Many of the doctors whom they consulted neglected that desire. The physicians came up with new tests and applied new treatments, but without positive results. In treating these kinds of patients, two mistakes were committed. First, the physicians did not have in their mental model the idea that climate affects people. Having no conception of this as a causative factor, they could not conceive of a solution.

<u>Case 1</u>. Mrs. Austin, fifty-six years old. Five years ago, she moved to Florida from Ohio. Since then, she has suffered from stuffiness in the chest, water retention, and a sensation that her head was held in a tight band. She felt ill. On the surface, this appears to be a very simple case. But Mrs. Austin suffered. She was acutely aware that this climate was not good for her, because each time she visited her grandchildren in California, her symptoms completely disappeared.

When I examined Mrs. Austin, I found that her pulse was rolling and her tongue was pale with a slippery coating. In Chinese medicine, such a case presents a typical dampness syndrome. The therapeutic principle is to increase spleen energy and transform the dampness to make the energy move smoothly, which means to increase the body's metabolism of water and so dry the internal environment. By this means, the patient's tolerance for humidity and damp will significantly improve.

After two months of acupuncture and Chinese herbal medicine treatment, Mrs. Austin's energy moved smoothly inside her body and her symptoms simply disappeared. The key to achieving this outcome was the concept of shaping the body to deal with the environment.

Case 2. Mrs. Lambert, sixty-four years old. She consulted me because of ankle edema, which was a pityable edema. She had undergone almost all the tests she could be given and had even consulted the Mayo Clinic in Jacksonville. Still, no diagnosis could be made. Mrs. Lambert herself observed that she should not live in Florida, because all her complaints began when she moved to Florida and when she goes away, her symptoms go away. This is not coincidental. However, Mrs. Lambert feels she has no choice. All the members of her family live in Florida, and her husband loves Florida weather.

Seeing no other way to go, Mrs. Lambert decided to try alternative medicine, and appeared in my office requesting treatment. Her pulse was rolling, her tongue was slippery. In Chinese medicine, her suffering is easily diagnosed as damp syndrome with spleen Qi deficiency. Treatment is very simple: increase spleen Qi (energy) and drain the damp from her body with acupuncture and Chinese herbal medicine formulae.

After two months treatment, Mrs. Lambert's symptoms completely disappeared. Some might say that is not a very challenging case, nonetheless, the patient endured a great deal of suffering for which modern western medicine offered no treatment. Chinese medicine, on the other hand, was very easy and very effective.

American medical practice needs to consider geographic factors. Then we can create—or at least implant—some effective techniques into our health-care system. Also, at least we can suggest that the patient live somewhere suitable for her/his body constitution.

Time and Seasons

In accordance with the same principle, people are affected by time and seasons. In some cases, a patient's symptoms will coalesce at certain times, otherwise that patient has no problem at all. Many cases illustrate this. For example, most chronic bronchitis is worse during the cold, winter season. Arthritis patients are worse during humid, rainy seasons. Patients with cardiovascular disease often get their attacks close to midnight.

This conception of Time has long been well recognized in Chinese medicine. The Time pattern was established when Yin-Yang theory and Five Elements theory (aspects of ancient Chinese philosophy) were incorporated into Chinese medicine. Daytime—and associated diseases—belongs to Yang. Nighttime—along with related diseases—belongs to Yin. Diseases related to Yang deficiency will worsen during Yin time. For example: the heart is a Yang organ, and during the Yin time (nighttime), Yang is under more stress. This is why heart patients are always worse at night.

The seasons and even the hours of the day were classified with respect to the elements and various internal organs. Spring belongs to the liver. Summer belongs to the heart. Late-summer belongs to the spleen. Autumn belongs to the lungs. Winter belongs to the kidneys. As very clearly described in the *Nei Jung* (one of the Classic Chinese Medical Books), different diseases attack people in different seasons. A distinguished and very practical theory evolved for treating and preventing disease according to different seasons and times of day. A famous historic case occurred in China in 1955 when epidemic encephalitis B occurred at Shijiazhuang. Relatively high curative effects were obtained by using Chinese medical herbs, primarily Gypsum decoction, which was prescribed by a well-known Chinese doctor, Pu Fuzhou, after he had gone to the epidemic area and observed the patients.

In 1956, epidemic encephalitis B occurred in the Beijing area. The same prescription was adopted, but patients failed to respond. The doctors changed their therapeutic strategies. Recognizing that the season was different, they added four other aromatic herbs to eliminate the damp/turbid effects of the prescription. The results were striking and the epidemic was controlled. Clearly: although the diseases appeared to be the same, their epidemic localities and seasons of onset were different. At Shijiazhuang encephalitis B occurred in the summer when the weather was hot and dry; in Beijing, it occurred during the late-summer/pre-autumn season when the weather was humid and damp because of an unbroken spell of rainfall. Consequently, they should not have been treated in the same way.

Case 3. Mr. Jiang, thirty-eight years old. He had a very interesting disease. For the past four years, he had suffered attacks of high fever, which began in mid-February. Each time Mr. Jiang suffered an acute episode, he ended up in hospital for infusion and heavy dosages of antibiotics over two- or three-week periods. According to his own description he went to hell once a year. After the most recent episode, he was totally exhausted. Otherwise, Mr. Jiang was a very strong man without complaint.

I saw him during the summer. He wanted me to help him to get rid of his problem. His pulse was wiry and his tongue was normal. A wiry pulse means liver Qi stagnation, but by itself is not sufficient evidence for a diagnosis. Considering that Mr. Jiang's problem fit the spring season (a liver-dominant period), my diagnosis was Liver Qi stagnation with liver deficiency. In the spring, liver Qi is normally strong enough to manage the whole body, but because Mr. Jiang's liver energy was weak, it could not carry out its responsibility, and allowed the invading pathogens to cause high fever. I prescribed Bupleurum Decoction to increase and to regulate his liver energy spring, which successfully cured his problem. The patient has had no episode of fever for the past three years.

Because diseases are associated with different times of day, treatments must also differ. Different organs dominate different times during the twenty-four hours of a day. Each organ dominates two hours. The gall-bladder dominates from 1 to 2 A.M.; the liver from 3 to 4 A.M., and so on. The development of modern chronology has provided a great deal of scientific data to explain this basic theory of Chinese medicine. Nonetheless, modern medical practice does not incorporate this concept, and so many cases cannot be properly treated.

> Case 4. Mrs. Showman, fifty-four years old. For seven years she had suffered from chronic hepatitis B. Most of the time, she was in a relative steady condition. Recently, she visited my office because of early morning sickness. Every morning around 3 to 4 A.M., she woke up with sweating and hot flushes, and chest oppression. She had undergone cardiovascular tests and hormone therapy without result. Obviously, the patient suffered neither a heart problem, nor a post-menopause syndrome. Her pulse was wiry and her tongue pale. The time of the attacks was a liver dominate time, so the diagnosis was liver Qi deficiency. I prescribed Bu Zhong Yi Qi Tang, a decoction to increase the middle Jiao[2] energy. After using that medicine for one week, Mrs. Showman's symptoms were completely controlled.

In these cases, the theoretical framework of medical analysis was more important than the concrete technique itself. Given the correct philosophical theory, the relative modality can be developed or established.

The Body Is a Single Inseparable Unit

—In the current biomedical model, to treat one problem is to cause a new problem.

In Chinese medical theory, the human body is an integral whole in which all organs and tissues have correspondences with one another. Normal physiological homeostasis is based on the perfect coordination of each organ with each other organ. Chinese medical philosophy aims to restore: balance or harmonization by treating the disease holistically. Neglecting this principle when treating patients invites disaster. In Chinese medicine, treating liver disease always entails using some herbal medicine to take care of the spleen/stomach system (the digestion system) in order to prevent the liver disease from affecting the spleen/stomach. In treating any kind of disease, one must know and care about the patient's stomach Qi, must be certain the patient can absorb the nutrient, must be certain that the patient will be able to have a good life, and live independently after recovering from the disease.

Because of the interrelationship between the lung and large intestine, when treating asthma patients, we take care of the large intestine at the same time and insure that the patient has a normal bowel movement, thereby allowing the respiratory system to gain the maxim benefit from the treatment. The interrelationship between the heart and kidney is emphasized in treating insomnia patients. Treating cardiovascular disease most often requires treating the stomach. Cardiologists are often puzzled by how a stomach problem can trigger palpitations, extra beats, or atrial fibrillations. Modern medicine knows nothing about these interrelationships, and by neglecting or ignoring them allows many unnecessary disasters to occur.

Case 5. Mr. Freeman, fifty-five years old. Three years ago Mr. Freeman consulted me about ascites due to post hepatitis B liver cirrhosis. He recovered very well with only Chinese herbal medicine treatment, and for more than two years, his liver profile remained in a normal range, with no ascites. Three months ago he hurt his back due to some improper work and wanted me to treat him for severe low back pain. I performed three sessions of acupuncture. His back pain was relieved by 50%, but I was not satisfied with the result. I suggested further examination by his medical doctor to confirm the diagnosis, never imagining how catastrophic that would be.

Mr. Freeman consulted a physician, who performed MRI and many other tests. The diagnosis was lumbar degeneration. The patient was put on coumodin and one pain killer, which caused severe subcutaneous bleeding, and his hemoglobin dropped to three. Mr. Freeman had a convulsive attack. Twelve units of transfused blood barely kept him alive. Finally Mr. Freeman left the hospital and quickly came to visit me. His back pain remained the same. However, he now had a huge hematoma in his back, and his liver situation had continued. Having no choice, I again put him on herbal medicine. Now he still has almost no back pain, and has returned to his normal life.

This is a typical case that happens almost every day. The modern medical model treated his pain, but forgot his liver situation, and forgot his blood platelet count and coagulation time. Such disasters can easily be avoided. I mention this case not to criticize the physician, but rather to criticize the medical system.

Case 6. Mr. Smith, seventy-three years old. He visited my office because of severe back pain. After three back surgeries, he collapsed. He could not walk and could not play golf anymore. Before these many surgeries, he had back pain, but he could still walk and play golf. He was very depressed. Mr. Smith was very weak and had cardiovascular disease and indigestion. His body might tolerate back surgery once, but no way could handle the second and third in a one-year period. The patient would get more benefits from surgery, had the surgeon considered the situation of the other organs, avoided traumatic therapy, and instead sought to improve the patient's general condition and increase his pain threshold.

Case 7. Mr. Kepler, seventy-five years old. In September 1995, after previously consulting sixteen other physicians, he visited my office as a last resort. His major complaint was severe cough. He had been coughing all day and all night for two months, could not sleep, and was losing weight fast. His cough began after heart bypass surgery two months earlier. Mr. Kepler was frustrated, and claimed that he would rather die than live this way, with no quality of life and so much suffering. Mr. Kepler was very fragile and weak. The bypass surgery may have cured his heart, but it created another disease even worse than his heart problem. While the technique for heart surgery is very sophisticated, and has allowed many people to survive, in this case it was a failure. The surgeon did not comprehensively evaluate the patient, and neglected the patient's weak lung condition; the surgery caused bronchial spasms and respiratory failure. Luckily, Mr. Kepler's exhaustive cough was cured in two months through acupuncture and herbal medicine.

Case 8. Mr. Robinson, fifty-six years old. A very nice man from Canada, Mr. Robinson had been diagnosed with lung cancer. He did not die of cancer, but from heart failure due to heavy dosages of chemotherapy. I mention him because he was a good man. His death also reminds us of the importance of conceptualizing the body as an inseparable unity.

How can we treat cancer and forget the heart, or other organs? It only causes more trouble for the patient. How many cancer patients have died from conventional therapy rather than from cancer? Why are so many cancer patients afraid of conventional treatments? We think that patients have been helped when, as a matter of fact, they suffer more and their survival rates are not significantly improved—not to mention the expense of chemotherapy and the related tests. Some have observed—and I agree with them—that the problem is the framework of our modern medical model.

The deficiency or shortcomings of this conceptual framework is shown in dealings with elderly patients. Most of the time, elderly patients do not suffer from only a single disease. A patient suffering from hypertension, for example, may at the same time suffer from diabetes or stomach ulcer or more. More than a dozen different medications are often prescribed and consumed every day by such patients! The human body has not been treated like an integral organ unit, but rather, like a machine into which medications are mechanically inserted with the blind faith that they will find their own ways to work on the different problems. Both doctor and patient are confused: neither knows which medications are essential, which are not, or even which side effect is coming from which drug. The patient's health gets worse and worse. We cannot blame the physicians. We have to blame their medical training.

Many patients who come to my office are very sick. They tell me that they faithfully take the prescription drugs but do not get any better. I suggest they discuss with their physician whether it's possible to stop all medications for a while and observe what happens. Many patients *even stop* taking massive dosages of drugs before they consult their physicians, and they feel better right away.

By contrast, Chinese medicine emphasizes interrelation and balance among the organs. The cause is determined through a comprehensive analysis of all the symptoms taken together as a whole. Each prescription is based on an entire "SYNDROME"—not only on separate symptoms. The cause is treated, and formulae of medicinal herbs simultaneously regulate the related organs to bring them into a new balance. The major principle is not to treat aggressively, but to regulate and harmonize the body by means of the body's own healing processes.

Case 9. Mr. Kennedy, eighty years old. He suffered severe insomnia, and had had no sleep at all since a prostate biopsy procedure 45 days earlier. He had been taking about 4 pills per day of Ambin, which had done nothing for his sleep. He was devastated, had no energy, and slight ankle edema. He also took two additional medications for his cardiovascular problem. Mr. Kennedy did not believe in alternative medicine, but he felt that at this moment he had no other choice. When I saw Mr. Kennedy, his complexion was flushed, his eyes were baggy and swollen; he was tired and frustrated. His heart pulse was very thin. The tip of his tongue was very red. He also complained of very dry mouth and lips.

My diagnosis was heart Yin Deficiency, and the major concern was to tonify the heart Yin. I prescribed an herbal formula combined with acupuncture to increase his heart Yin. He responded very quickly to this treatment, and in two weeks, he could use one Ambin to sleep 7 hours every day. All his symptoms were gone; he was able to play golf again. Why his heart Yin deficiency? It is most often caused by overdoses of diuretics which create a state of near dehydration.

Case 10. Mr. Brown, ninety-three years old. His major complaint was diarrhea and weight loss. He had been passing watery diarrhea, with undigested food in 6–8 bowel movements per day for 8 months. His height was 6'3", his weight was 120 lb.—very slim.

"Conventional medicine and gastroentrologists have done all they can," his wife told me. I gave him a physical examination. No malignancy was apparent. His heart pulse and lung pulse were very weak. In Chinese medicine, we claim that the small intestine is related to heart, and the lung related to the large intestine. Food cannot be absorbed when there is no heart fire to help fermentation. The heart dominates the whole body Yang. Now his heart Yang deficiency was the key—nothing was related to his gastrointestinal system.

I prescribed a Chinese herbal formula Yang Xin Tang (Decoction to Tonify Heart). In three days, his bowel movements were down to 2 to 3 times per day, almost formed. In two weeks, his bowel movements were back to normal, his energy had improved and he had gained back 12 lb. If I had treated only his gastrointestinal system, there would have been no result, because heart Yang deficiency was the root pathology in his disease.

Balance and Harmony Is the Final Goal of the Treatment

—Overdoing is the major cause of medical crisis in modern medicine.

In Chinese medicine, we emphasize balance between Yin and Yang, and harmony among all the internal organs. Disease is the breakdown of this balance and harmony. To treat the disease is to recover the original balance.

In the modern medicine model, we create and use many strong drugs and therapies to treat diseases. We forget the concept of balance and harmony in the body. In curing one problem, we often create another and place the patient in an unending vicious circuit. We need to train our doctors to understand this principle—not only to know how to treat by getting rid of disease, but also how to promote life. A very simple and familiar example is the overdosage of antibiotics to kill one bacterium, and while healing this infection, the balance of bacterial strains is disturbed, and yeast infection always follows. In clinical practice, we meet so many elderly patients often taking three or four antibiotics at the same time for urinary tract infection. And even with this very heavy dosage, they continue to suffer from the infection. What has happened is that the over-use of the drugs has brought the body further and further away from its balanced state. We have made the patient worse.

For chronic disease, we need an accurate diagnosis and low dosages to invigorate the body's healing system and stimulate it to achieve its own balance. The problem lies in not respecting the ability of the body to heal itself. We try to kill bacteria, to kill viruses, to kill organisms, to kill cancer cells. Why not think more about how and why these evils invade and attack the body? Chinese medicine emphasizes that the cause of pathogenic invasion is the body's weakness. If the body is strengthened and balanced, bacteria/virus and tumor cells will have no opportunity to grow. But we neglect this, knowing only how to kill with strong drugs. In the treatment of cancer, survival rates have shown no significant improvement in the last 30 years. This does not parallel the great advancements in modern biomedical techniques. Why? We can arrive at a clear answer only if we consider the question from the perspective of philosophy or methodology.

So many new chemotherapy drugs have been developed for killing tumor cells. But what do we do to balance the body and increase the body energy? Nothing. In Chinese medicine, we do not have these powerful drugs, but the medicines are more natural and more easily accepted by patient's body. Tumors and cancers are caused by imbalances among various internal organs—not only by imbalance in the affected organs. In lung cancer, for example, spleen deficiency forms phlegm, and liver involvement causes energy stagnation. Lung cancer is a compensatory reaction to poor spleen and liver performance. Therefore: to treat lung cancer, we should focus on transforming the phlegm and regulating the liver energy in order to recover the balance among these three organs. The treatment is gentle, but it works. Often it works much better than the conventional cancer therapy.

Case 11. Mrs. Mitchell, seventy-two years old. After being diagnosed with lung cancer (adendocarcinoma), she was put on chemotherapy. After two sessions, the patient collapsed; her body was very weak, bone marrow depressed. She could not tolerate the chemotherapy at all. She was then put on Prednisone and Radiation therapy. After two sessions, she had a compression fracture, and suffered horribly from severe pain. She claimed she would rather die than continue with this therapy. I fully understood why this patient sought alternative therapy.

At the time Mrs. Mitchell became my patient, she was very weak, with a lot of pain in her upper back and rib cage, severe depression, and shortness of breath (she also had emphysema). I used gentle acupuncture to relieve her pain and depression, and a Chinese herbal formula to increase her spleen energy, regulate liver energy. Gradually she gained more energy and became stronger without chemo and radiation therapy. Her lung cancer became so stable that her MRIs have shown no growth or metastasis in two years. The tumor size even began to diminish. If we could incorporate this concept into our daily clinical practice, we could achieve many more beneficial effects.

As modern medical techniques progress, the branches of medicine are becoming more and more specialized. One patient may have five or six doctors, each doctor prescribes different drugs. Lack of communication and harmonization among the doctors creates a plethora of problems. How can they promote balance in the body? How can they help their patients to balance the organs and achieve a cure? We have the general practitioner, who should regularly respond to and communicate with the patient's varied specialists about the medications and therapies. But in fact, most of them fail to do this job. Often you see a patient taking more than ten different drugs, some of which counteract each other. The patients have paid for expensive medicines that only make them more sick. Balance and harmonization means not only harmonizing the patient's body; it also means harmonizing the doctor and patient. Actually, that is another big topic.

Ethics and Multi-dimensional Thinking

—Caring and flexible/multiple treatments can boost the body's natural healing process to heal pernicious disease.

Many complaints are heard about practitioners' attitudes and manners in modern medicine. Doctors do not spend enough time with patients, and they rush the patient too much. And it is very difficult to get appointments when you really need them. Or they do not take the patient seriously, and so on.

Medical ethics has been a big topic since the very beginning of medical practice. In Chinese medicine, it is the first required class that a medical school student takes. Many ancient famous doctors had excellent descriptions of ethics. Confucian philosophy, the main essence of Chinese medical ethics, requires that doctors treat patients as they would treat their parents or siblings. In Confucianism, parents and the emperor held the highest status. You were not allowed to neglect, abandon, or mistreat them. That was the law. How you treated your parents was the standard for judging your personality—whether you were a good or bad person. So: if doctors treated their patients as their relatives, there would be no problem about medical ethics.

In the Tang Dynasty (618–906 A.D.), the very famous doctor Sun Simiao[3] wrote a beautiful statement of medical ethics, which is almost the same as the medical ethics oath of the Greek physician Hippocrates, written four hundred years later. Sun's code of ethics was passed from generation to generation in Chinese medical schools. Hippocrates' oath was consigned to history.

In the U.S. I have met many mothers who were seeking an alternative to vaccination for their children. I found this phenomenon very surprising. With the great advance of modern science, how is it that so many people have come to want to avoid vaccination, which has been so successful in preventing deadly infectious disease? The parents are very certain that they do not want their children vaccinated. If I advise them to get their children vaccinated, they may become angry with me. But my medical ethics and my heart forces me to persuade them to let their children be vaccinated. Some of them even said, "I came here for something new—otherwise why am I here?" I patiently educate them about the importance of vaccinations for the child's future. Most of them listen to me and get their children vaccinated.

The underlying problem is our physicians—particularly some doctors who claim to do alternative medicine, and who want to please their patients even to the extent of neglecting basic science. By the way, originally vaccination technique was invented in ancient China. As physicians we have to do things from our heart if we are concerned about doing good for our patients. Medical practice is not a business. We cannot disobey our medical ethics and basic common sense to attract patients, and we cannot take the patient as our client for business' sake. But in this country, medical practice has becoming a big business. I have no idea how to solve this problem.

For many cancer patients' treatment, the medical routine is MRI and biopsy for diagnosis, then surgery, then chemo- or radiation-therapy, and finally the patient is exhausted or tired to death—rarely recovered. Here I quote the *New England Journal of Medicine* (1997; 336:1569–74) "Despite decades of basic and clinical research and trials of promising new therapies, cancer remains a major cause of morbidity and mortality. . . . The war against cancer is far from over. Observed changes in mortality are due to early detection. The effect of new treatments for cancer on mortality has been largely disappointing."

Ask oncologists, how much do they trust this routine therapy? Have they seen whether this therapy works or not? If their own parent suffers cancer, are they willing to put them on this routine therapy? I doubt it. But treating cancer is big money business. And insurance companies will pay for this therapy.

Case 12. Mrs. Washington, forty-seven years old. She is an electronic engineer, and very intelligent. In March 1996 she was diagnosed through biopsy with a very malignant breast carcinoma. Her oncologist strongly suggested removing the mass through surgery while the cancer was still in its early stage—the best time to have surgery. But Mrs. Washington refused surgery. She came to my office for alternative therapy.

For her situation, what should I do? That is a big dilemma for me. To suggest that she go back for surgery? To accept her as a patient and treat her with Chinese medicine exclusively? In comparison to the conventional therapy for cancer, Chinese medicine works very well, but it is very slow, working through boosting the body natural healing system to achieve a cure. It takes time. Surgically removing the mass could win time for the Chinese herbal medicine treatment. In the early stage of cancer treatment, if surgery is available, it is obviously correct to do! For Mrs. Washington, surgery was the right thing to do. I have seen many breast cancer patients survive and live very well after the early stage cancer was surgically removed.

So I advised her to return for surgery. But she was very convinced about what she wanted and what she was doing. In general, she was deeply disappointed with modern medicine. She was afraid of conventional therapy. She told me what happened to her friend and neighbor, a 49-year-old man. During an annual physical examination, enlarged lymph nodes were found in his left neck. His doctor suggested a biopsy, which confirmed non-Hodgkin's lymphoma. Then he was put on chemotherapy, became exhausted, caught pneumonia, and died—all in a period of two months. Mrs. Washington thought that if her friend had not taken the rough treatment of chemotherapy, he might still be alive. I pushed her very hard, but finally gave up. She has her instincts. We have to respect her feelings. I accepted her as a patient for treatment with Chinese herbal medicine and dietary regulation.

Fortunately, without surgery, chemotherapy, and radiation therapy, she is still in good shape. The breast tumor is slightly larger. But she feels fine, without any metastasis and her cancer antigen is in the normal range. Her weight has remained almost the same.

If our oncologists can get their patient's trust and get the surgery done, then the patient will receive the greatest benefit from the combination with Chinese herbal medicine treatment. As a Chinese medicine practitioner, I can more easily fulfill my role. Patients will take less risk. The oncologists should rethink their status and differentiate individual cases: do not treat all cancer patients with one invariant medical model and routine.

The cases I have described are real cases. These types of problems are an incredible phenomenon, and you can encounter them every day in your practice. What do you want to do—as an oncologist, as a physician? We must change, we must improve our performance. My thinking is to construct another, a better medical model: one that would introduce Chinese medical philosophies and ethics into the current medical healthcare system. As to *how* to integrate the Chinese medical philosophies into the current medical model: many things need to be discussed. It cannot happen in one or two days. But it is essential to improve the quality of medical practice and create a better medical model that would greatly benefit our people.

Summary

This paper proposes a new holistic medical model that would introduce fundamental principles of Chinese medicine into current medical practice, thus strengthening the effectiveness of conventional medicine, while at the same time addressing some of its shortcomings. The new medical model will involve multi-dimensional thinking and will adopt varied therapeutic modalities, allowing patients to receive maximum benefit from modern medical techniques.

The main points discussed in this paper center around 1) the necessity to recognize the relationship between the human body and natural factors such as weather, locality, time; 2) the need to conceptualize and treat the body as a single inseparable unit in which all organ systems are interrelated; 3) the value of emphasizing balance and harmony (rather than the simple elimination of disease) as a goal of treatment; and 4) the promise of reevaluating assumptions about medical ethics and the relationship between doctor and patient.

As what I mentioned above how to integrate Chinese Medical philosophies into current medical model means to go into detail and submitting another paper. At least I think we need to educate medical students at university level about these two existing healthcare systems. Only then are we able to accomplish what I call the best medical model for the well-being of every person.

Acknowledgment: Great thanks to Dr. Carolyn Bloomer, (Ph.D.) for editing this paper in her busy schedule. Thanks also to my colleague Dr. Helga Wall-Apelt (M.D.) for her great support. Without their help and encouragement, this book would not be available.

Notes

1. All the cases mentioned in this paper are actual cases. Patients' names have been changed for the purpose of confidentiality.
2. Middle Jiao is a physiological terminology in Chinese Medicine, which indicates the middle portion of the body, especially for spleen and stomach.
3. Sun Si Miao, who was the author of *Qian Jin Fang* (The Formulas Worth of Thousand Tons of Gold).

Appendix
A Chronology of Chinese Medicine

Prehistory (c. 30th to 18th centuries B.C.). Reigns of the "celestial emperors," who taught the Chinese people the arts and sciences of agriculture, music, handicrafts, writing, and so on. Among them was Shen Nong, inventor of agriculture, who created the basis for the first pharmacopoeia, and Huang Di, the inventor of medicine.

—c. 19th–13th centuries B.C.
—Egyptian, Babylonian, Vedic, and Hebrew writings on medicine

Shang Dynasty (1765–1122 B.C.)

Later medicinal books refer to herbal treatments dating from this dynasty. Names of diseases were inscribed on oracle bones that have been found in tombs dating from this era.

11th–6th centuries B.C.
References in the later books *Shi Jing*, *Shan Hai Jing*, and *Zhou Li* points to theories current during this era concerning the relationship of epidemic diseases to the weather and the seasons.

Zhou Dynasty (1121–249 B.C.)

6th century B.C.
 Appearance of Daoism.
 References to connection between rabies and dogs behaving in strange ways.
 The doctor Yi He treated the King of Jin State. He was the first to use the theory of "Six Evil Qi" to explain the pathogenesis of disease.
 The famous doctor Bian Que is born.

5th century B.C.–3rd century A.D.
 Zu Bei Mai Jiu Jing—thought to be the first document about meridian and collateral theory.
 Huang Di Nei Jing ("Internal Classic Cannon of the Yellow Emperor")
  —5th–1st centuries B.C.—Hippocrates and beginnings of Greek medicine

4th century B.C.
 Confucius

Warring States Period (248–222 B.C.)

3rd century B.C.—3rd century A.D.)
 First clinical use of case recording and study documents.
 Huang Di Ba Shi Yi Nan Jing ("Yellow Emperor's Book of 81 Difficult Questions")
 First application of medicine via patch.

Han Dynasty (206 B.C.–220 A.D.)

1st century B.C.
Buddhism.
Li Guo Zhu, a doctor of the royal family, reedited and corrected the medical books preserved by the government. There were seven books in medical theory, eleven books about herbal medicine and formulas.

1st century A.D.
Shen Nong Ben Cao Jing ("Yellow Emperor's Pharmacopoeia").
The folk doctor Po Wong wrote *Zhen Jing*, about acupuncture, and *Zhen Mai Fa*, about pulse diagnosis.
Famous doctor Guo Yu.
—1st century A.D.—Galen, famous Greek surgeon

2nd century A.D.
Hua Tuo performed open abdominal surgery with orally administered anesthetic. He advocated the physical exercise therapy called *Qi Gong*.
Zhang Zhong Jing wrote *Shang Han Za Bing Lun*, to establish the medical therapeutic principle of differentiation of syndrome according to Six Channels.
Evidence of Tibetan doctors using a particular plant oil as an anti-bleeding medicine.

3rd century A.D.
Wang Shu He wrote *Mai Jing* ("Pulse Diagnosis").
First published case studies.

Jin Dynasty (265–419 A.D.)

265 A.D.–341 A.D.
First text on acupuncture and moxibustion, by Huang Fu Mi.
—4th–5th centuries—Christian hospitals appeared in Rome

South and North Dynasties (420–589 A.D.)

420 A.D.–479 A.D.
Lei Gong Pao Zhi Lun, the first book on pharmaceutical technique, or how to prepare herbs before they were taken as medicine.

5th century
Gong Qing Xuan wrote *Liu Juan Zi Gui Yi Fang*, the first book about surgical diseases.

562 A.D.
Wu Ren Zhi Cong brought *Ming Tang Tu*, a 60-volume Chinese medical encyclopedia, to Japan.

Sui Dynasty (589–618 A.D.)

608 A.D.
Japan sent pharmacists to China to study Chinese herbal medicine.

610 A.D.
Cao Yuan Fang and others compiled *Zhu Bing Yuan Hou Lun* ("Etiology and Manifestation of Many Diseases"), which was the first extant text on pathology.
Recognition of athlete's foot.

Tang Dynasty (619–907 A.D.)

7th century
 Vaccination against smallpox.

624 A.D.
 The Royal Medical Institute taught medicine according to different specialties.

640 A.D.
 First description of psychiatric diseases by Sun Si Miao.
 Recognition of diabetes symptoms and signs.

659 A.D.
 Su Jing and his collegues were ordered to compile the first national pharmacopedia, *Xin Xiu Ben Cao* (new edition of the Shen Nong Pharmacopedia).

581 A.D.–682 A.D.
 Sun Xi Miao wrote *Qian Jin Yao Fang* ("A Thousand Golden Formulas") and *Qian Jin Yi Fang* ("A Thousand Golden Supplementary Formulas").
 Night blindness treated with liver.

612 A.D.–714 A.D.
 Meng She wrote *Shi Liao Ben Cao* ("Medicines for Food and Medical Use").
—8th century—Arabian doctors revived Greek medical texts; Europe languished in the Middle Ages

713 A.D.–714 A.D.
 Chen Zang Qi wrote *Ben Cao Shi Yi* ("Collection of the Missed Medicines by the Current Pharmacopedia").

752 A.D.
  Wang Tao wrote *Wai Tai Mi Yao* ("Essential Secrets from the Master's Podium")
  First description of cataract surgery.

762 A.D.
  Wang Bing reedited and annotated the classic *Huang Di Nei Jing Su Wei*.

841 A.D.–846 A.D.
  Li Dao Ren wrote *Xian Shou Li Shang Xu Duan Mi Fang* ("Secret Formulas and Techniques for Disposing of Injury and Bone Fracture").

847 A.D.–859 A.D.
  Jiu Yin wrote *Jing Xiao Chan Bao* ("Treasured Techniques for Menstruation and Delivery"), the earliest gynecological book in Chinese medical history.
     —896—Persian doctors identify measles and smallpox.

8th–9th Century
  The special pharmaceutic chemical technique for preparing medicines was spread to Arab countries.

Song Dynasty (960–1279 A.D.)

982–992 A.D.
  Wang Huai Yi and others wrote *Tai Ping Sheng Hui Fang* (Peaceful and Charity Formulas), which was the earliest and largest book of medicinal formulas.

10th century
  Theories of Li Xue and Xin Xue.

1026 A.D.

Wang Wei Yi wrote *Tong Ren Shu Xuan Zhen Jiu Tu Jing* ("Graphic Book of Acupuncture and Moxibustion Points in Bronzed Statues"). The next year, Wang Wei Yi designed and cast the famous bronze statues used for the study of acupuncture.

1057 A.D.

Song government established the Department of Reediting Classical Medical Books, to publish the classical medical and pharmacopedia books.

1076 A.D.

The Royal Medical Institutes built the first national pharmacy.

1086 A.D.

Han Zhi He wrote *Shang Han Wei Zhi* ("The Delicate Essences in Febrile Disease Caused by Cold").

1093 A.D.

Dong Ji wrote *Xiao Er Ban Zhen Bei Ji Fang Lun* ("Discussions on Rash and Skin Spots in Pediatrics").

1098 A.D.

Yang Zi Jian wrote *Shi Chan Lun* ("Ten Topics on Baby Delivery"), which was the first Obstetrics book in Chinese history.

—11th century—Avicenna published comprehensive medical encyclopedia

11th century

A formula for inducing labor was discovered.

1100 A.D.
Shang Han Zong Bing Lun ("The General Discussion on Febrile Disease Caused by Cold").

1102–1106 A.D.
Cun Zhen Tu ("The True Illustrated Anatomy") by Yang Jie, according to his observations from the dissection of corpses.

1107 A.D.
Chen Shi Wen and his collegues wrote *Tai Ping Hui Min He Ji Ju Fang*, which is one of the most extensive formulas books ever written. Zhu Hong wrote *Lei Zheng Huo Ren Shu* ("Categorization of Syndrome to Rescue the People"), which was a very important clinical book.

1116 A.D.
Kou Zong Bi wrote *Ben Cao Yan Yi* ("The Extension of Materia Medica").

1119 A.D.
Yan Xiao Zhong collected Qian Yi's clinical experience compiled into *Xiao Er Yao Zheng Zhi Jue* ("Medicine and Clinical Manifestation in Pediatrics"), which was respected as the first specialized text on pediatrics in Chinese medical history.
—12th century—Maimonides the Physician

Yuan Dynasty (1206–1368)

13th century
First steroid is manufactured.

1217–1221 A.D.
Zhang Cong Zheng wrote *Ru Men Shi Qi* ("Confucian School to Take Care of Parents"), a very practical clinical book,

in which the purgative/diaphoretic therapeutic theories were developed in detail.

1220 A.D. (South Song, Jia Ding 13th year)
Wang Zhi Zhong wrote *Zhen Jiu Zi Sheng Jing* ("Productive Book of Acupuncture & Moxibustion"), which was a clinical manual for acupuncture and moxibustion.

1226 A.D.
Wen Ren Shi Nian wrote *Bei Ji Jiu Fa* ("Moxibustion Technique for Emergencies").

1237 A.D.
Zhen Zhi Ming wrote *Fu Ren Da Quan Liang Fang* ("General Health Formulas for Women"). This is the first gynecological book in Chinese medical history.

1247 A.D.
Song Ci wrote *Xi Yuan Lu* ("The Recording of Reversing Misjudged Criminal Cases"), which was the first text on forensic medicine.

1263 A.D.
The first comprehensive surgical text appeared.
   —1270—physicians in Cairo described circulation.

1294 A.D.
Cao Shi Rong wrote *Huo You Xin Shu* ("New Book to Rescue Babies"), an advanced pediatrics book for dealing with emergency cases.
   —1302—First legal autopsy performed in Europe, in Bologna.

1343 A.D.
Wei Yi Lin wrote *Shi Yi De Xiao Fang* ("Effective Formula & Technique for All Generations of Doctors"), an authoritative book on traumatology and orthopedics.

1348 A.D.
>Tuberculosis identified.
>>—1377—Quarantine introduced for infectious diseases.

Ming Dynasty (1368–1662)

1442
>Leng Qian wrote *Xiu Ling Yao Zhi* ("The Key for Longevity").

1443
>Royal Health Institute of Ming published the *Tong Ren Shu Xue Zhen Jiu Tu Jing* and cast new bronze acupuncture models.
>—1536—Paracelsus wrote treatise on surgical technique. 15th century—Leonardo da Vinci produced detailed anatomical drawings.

1540 A.D.
>Syphilis identified as spread by sexual contact.

1550
>Shen Zhi Wei wrote *Jie Wei Yuan Shu* ("The Techniques for Treating Leprosy").

1554
>Xue Ji wrote *Li Yang Ji Yao* ("The Key to Treating Dermatological Diseases").

1567–1572
>Vaccination technique was recorded as first used in the Tang Dynasty.
>>—1590—Invention of microscope.

1591
    Gao Lian wrote *Zui Sheng Ba Qian* ("Eight Principles for Preservation of Health").

1602–1608
    Wang Ken Tang wrote *Zhen Zhi Zhun Sheng* (The Standard for Diagnosis and Treatment).

1604
    Gong Yun Lin wrote *Xiao Er Tui Na Mi Zhi* ("Secret Massage Techniques for Use in Pediatrics").
        —1616—William Harvey wrote about blood circulation.

1617
    Chen Shi Gong wrote *Wai Ke Zheng Zong* ("The Standards of Surgical Technique and Medicinal Formulas").

1644
    Fu Ren Yu wrote *Shen Shi Yao Han* ("The Treasure for Vision"), the first specific text on ophthalmology.
        —1665—Robert Hooke described cells.
        1667—First blood transfusion.
        1673—van Leeuwenhoek described red corpuscles.
        1688—Cataract surgery with gold needle.
        1783—Digitalis identified as a cure for dropsy.
        1796—Jenner introduces vaccination.
        1819—Invention of stethoscope.

Qing Dynasty (1662–1911)

1822
    Qing government prohibited the practice of acupuncture and moxibustion in the Royal Health Institute.

1830

Wang Qing Ren wrote *Yi Lin Gai Cuo* ("Correcting the Mistakes in the Medical Forest"), which included anatomy knowledge and his own findings and clinical experiences.

—1831—Chloroform used for anaesthesia.

1844

Under pressure, the Qing government agreed to let Americans build clinics and churches in the coastal cities.

—1851—Invention of ophthalmoscope.

1851–1864

The government of Tainping Tian Guo (Peaceful Heaven Kingdom) built hospitals, sanitation facilities, and strictly prohibited the opium trade and outlawed prostitution.

—1882—Tuberculosis bacterium identified.
1889—Diabetes connected to pancreatic function.

1844–1948

British and Americans built many hospitals and medical schools in Macao, Xia Men, Ningbo, Shanghai, and Fuzhou.

1884

Tang Zong Hai wrote *Zhong Xi Hui Tong Yi Shu Wu Zhong* ("Five Books of Interpretation between Chinese and Western Medicine").

1901

Zheng Xiao Yan wrote *Shu Yi Yue Bain* ("The Compressed Edition of the Plague Caused by Rats").

—1901—Adrenaline identified.

Republic of China (1912–1948)

1914
Temporary government of Bei Yang (North Military Group) advocated ending Traditional Chinese Medicine.

1925
Guomindang (National Party) government prohibited course of Traditional Chinese Medicine in medical schools.
—1926—Anemia treated with liver.

1928
Mao Ze Dong, the Chairman of the Communist Party, advocated combining Chinese medicine with Western medicine to treat disease.

1929 (18th year of Min Guo)
"The Plan of Getting Rid of Old Medicine" advocated by Yu Yan was approved by the Guomindang government, resulting in striking workers in the medical and pharmaceutical fields.

1932
Discovery of asthma medicine ephedrine.

1936
The Guomindang government issued the "Law of Traditional Chinese Medicine."

1945–1947
Japanese invaders destroyed a bacteria manufacture company, which caused an outbreak of the plague.

People's Republic of China (1949–)

1949

The People's Republic of China established the Central Hygiene Administration.

1950

The Academy of Traditional Chinese Medicine and the University of Traditional Chinese Medicine were built in Beijing. Three other Traditional Chinese medicine schools were built in Guangzhou, Sichuan, and Shanghai.

1955

Most of the inner provinces have at least one Traditional Chinese Medical school.

1967–1977

The Cultural Revolution. Many teachers and doctors were sent to labor camps.

1977

National education and examination systems finally recovered completely. Medical schools selected students through a strict national examination.

1981

The postgraduate student system was recovered.

References

1. Eisenberg, D., M.D., Kessler, R.C., et al. "Unconventional Medicine in the United States. *New England Journal of Medicine* 328(4): 246–252, 1993.
2. Gerber, R., M.D. *Vibrational Medicine*—New choice for healing oneself. Santa Fe: Bear & Co., 1996.
3. Dossey, L., M.D. *Space, Time & Medicine*. Boston: Shambhala, 1985.
4. McDowell, B., and Andrew Weil, M.D.—"Championing Integrative Medicine," in *Alternative Complementary Therapies*. 1:8–13, 1994.
5. Arno, P., Ph.D. and K. Feiden. *Against the Odds—The Story of AIDS Drug Development, Politics & Profits*. New York: Harper Collins, 1992.
6. Liu, B. Q., Wang, Q. L. *Optimum Time for Acupuncture—A Collection of Traditional Chinese Chronotherapeutics*. Shangdong, China: Science & Technology Press, 1988.
7. Magner, L., *A History of Medicine*. New York: Marcel Dekker, Inc., 1992.
8. Porkert, M., M.D. *Chinese Medicine*. New York: An Owl Book, Henry Holt and Company, 1982.
9. Porkert, M., M.D. *The Essentials of Chinese Diagnostics*. Zurich, Switzerland: Chinese Medicine Publications, LTD, 1974.
10. Sun, Simiao. *Qian Jin Fang* (Medicinal Formulas Valued Thousands Tons of Gold). Beijing: Hua Xia Publisher, 1993.
11. Chen, Y.B. Deng, L.Y. and et al. *Dangdai Zhongguo Zhen Jiu Li Zheng Jing Yao* (The Collection of Excellent Acupuncture Clinical Case Studies). Tianjin: Science & Technique Press.
12. Zhang, Y.Q. ECIWO *Biology and Medicine:* A New Theory of Conquering Cancer and a Completely New Acupuncture Therapy. Nei Meng Gu People's Press.